House Officer
SERIES

Weiner and Levitt's Neurology

EIGHTH EDITION

Alexander Rae-Grant, M.D., F.R.C.P.(C.)
Neurological Institute,
Cleveland Clinic
Cleveland, Ohio

The House Officer Series is based on Weiner and Levitt's
Neurology for the House Officer, first published in 1973.

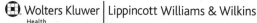

Wolters Kluwer | Lippincott Williams & Wilkins
Health
Philadelphia · Baltimore · New York · London
Buenos Aires · Hong Kong · Sydney · Tokyo

Acquisitions Editor: Frances DeStefano
Managing Editor: Leanne McMillan
Project Manager: Alicia Jackson
Senior Manufacturing Manager: Benjamin Rivera
Marketing Manager: Kimberly Schonberger
Design Coordinator: Terry Mallon
Cover Designer: Andrew Gatto
Production Service: International Typesetting and Composition

© 2008, by LIPPINCOTT WILLIAMS & WILKINS, a WOLTERS KLUWER business.
530 Walnut Street
Philadelphia, PA 19106 USA
LWW.com

Seventh Edition, © 2004 by Lippincott Williams & Wilkins, Sixth Edition © 1999 by Williams & Wilkins

Printed in the USA

Library of Congress Cataloging-in-Publication Data

Rae-Grant, Alexander.
   Weiner and Levitt's neurology/Alexander Rae-Grant—8th ed.
      p. ; cm.—(House officer series)
   Rev. ed. of: Neurology/Howard L. Weiner. 7th ed. c2004.
   Includes bibliographical references and index.
   ISBN-13: 978-0-7817-8154-1
   ISBN-10: 0-7817-8154-X
   1. Nervous system—Diseases—Handbooks, manuals, etc.   2.
Neurology—Handbooks, manuals, etc.   I. Weiner, Howard L. Neurology.   II.
Title.   III. Title: Neurology.   IV. Series.
   [DNLM: 1. Nervous System Diseases. 2. Neurologic Manifestations. WL 140
R134w 2007]
   RC355.W44 2007
   616.8—dc22

                                       2007047319

To purchase additional copies of this book, call our customer service department at **(800) 638-3030** or fax orders to **(301) 223-2320**. International customers should call **(301) 223-2300**.

Visit Lippincott Williams & Wilkins on the Internet: at LWW.com. Lippincott Williams & Wilkins customer service representatives are available from 8:30 am to 6 pm, EST.

                                                10 9 8 7 6 5 4 3 2 1

To the many students, residents, and fellows that Drs. Levitt, Weiner, and I have had the privilege of working with during our careers. To my wife Mary Bruce and my children who have been so supportive over the years. Finally to my colleagues and friends, Dr. Howard Weiner and Dr. Lawrence Levitt, who allowed me to participate in this wonderful endeavor.

Foreword

Osler once observed that attempting to learn medicine without a text reference can be likened to sailing off to sea without navigation equipment. Dr. Rae-Grant, in the latest edition of *Neurology for the House Officer*, provides the trainee with a small, pocket-sized reference that can be likened to the GPS navigation devices currently popular in automobiles.

Thirty-four years have elapsed since the first edition of this pocket marvel appeared. In his foreword to that edition Dr. H. Richard Tyler observed that the original offering was compiled from lecture notes by Dr. Weiner and Dr. Levitt, then residents in the Harvard Neurology program. The intent was for local consumption and distribution to students and house officers rotating on the Neurology services in the Harvard program. Since then seven editions have come and gone with distribution through the American market and several international translations.

The new eighth edition offers significant modification from previous versions with a new chapter on evidence-based neurology, a new glossary supplement, as well as therapeutic updates, where appropriate, together with a new set of references. Chapters have been revised to incorporate these changes.

Weiner and Levitt's Neurology is a "must have" for Neurology and Internal Medicine residents alike. As a pocket reference, it is unsurpassed.

Dr. Patrick Sweeney, MD, FACP
Neurological Institute,
Cleveland Clinic

About Dr. Sweeney: Dr. Sweeney is a long-time attending physician at the Cleveland Clinic and highly regarded for his leadership and teaching abilities. He was recently awarded the Alfred and Norma Lerner Humanitarian Award, Cleveland Clinic's most prestigious physician honor.

Foreword to the First Edition (1973)

Having spent my professional life in a teaching hospital with a steady stream of students, house officers, and residents, I have gradually become accustomed to the varying neurologic backgrounds of these young physicians.

The neurologist and the internist exhibit significant differences in approach. The internist is usually trained to think physiologically in terms of the meaning and cause of specific symptoms. The neurologist, on the other hand, brings to the patient encounter not only his history and physical examination but a special "neurologic examination." This special examination is designed more to answer the question "where is the lesion" than "what is wrong with the patient." The neurologist, therefore, can profit tremendously from a knowledge of neuroanatomy and neuro-physiology combined with a careful neurologic examination and appropriate evaluation.

In this country, most students and medical residents, general practitioners, and internists do not develop strong backgrounds in neurology. They therefore profit less from their neurologic endeavors than they might. Nevertheless, they are still required to care for patients with nervous system disorders and are often significantly insecure about treatment.

In attempting to deal with this problem, two of our most capable neurology residents, Howard L. Weiner, MD, and Lawrence P. Levitt, MD, began compiling notes from their lectures to small groups of students. This soon became source material for future reference. The demand for this material grew geometrically and was widely used by students and residents. The need for a practical manual was appreciated, and the authors began a more systematic approach to problems with which they were recurrently faced on the wards of a large teaching hospital. As fast as they could put the sections out, students, medical interns, and residents kept requesting them, and soon large numbers were being duplicated. The material was recognized for its practical and common sense approach to problems frequently encountered.

After 2 years of intense effort to gather constructive suggestions, find unmet needs, and weed out unimportant material, the authors have written this handbook.

It was originally planned for local use in our hospitals and given to students and residents rotating through the service. As requests for the handbook began to arrive from many areas, the need for wider circulation was appreciated. This need was translated into the decision to publish this handbook.

Since it has been so enthusiastically received by critical students and residents here, we believe it will meet the practical needs of young physicians elsewhere.

H. Richard Tyler, MD

About the Author

Alex Rae-Grant, MD, FRCP(C), is a staff neurologist at the Cleveland Clinic Foundation. He is the past president of the medical staff, Lehigh Valley Hospital, Allentown, Pennsylvania, and prior chief of the division of neurology, Lehigh Valley Hospital. A graduate of Yale University, he attended McMaster University Medical School in Ontario. He was a medical resident at Sunnybrook Hospital of the University of Toronto, and did his neurology training at the University of Western Ontario in London, Ontario. He co-wrote the past two editions of *Neurology for the House Officer* with Dr. Howard Weiner and Dr. Lawrence Levitt. He also co-edited *The 5-Minute Neurology Consult*.

Preface

It has been an honor to carry on the tradition of *Neurology for the House Officer* for this, its eighth edition. In this edition I have tried to fully update each chapter with new information on the diagnosis and treatment of neurologic disorders. At the same time I have tried to keep the style as conversational and readable as the prior editions that Drs. Weiner and Levitt initiated. I have inserted a new chapter on Evidence-Based Medicine in neurology, as well as a much-needed glossary of commonly used neurologic terms. I have updated some of the figures with the help of my son, Michael Rae-Grant. I have also tried to make the neurologic method of diagnosis more explicit in this edition. I referenced key changes in neurologic practice while continuing to highlight useful information for students of neurology. I have also referred to the levels of evidence for many therapeutic suggestions in line with changes in the field of medicine. Above all, I have continued the philosophic goal of this text: to provide an easily digestible text in neurology for those relatively new to the field. This text is not meant to be a compendium of all neurologic information, but rather a starting point for further inquiry that does not dampen the ardor of potential students of the field.

Alex D. Rae-Grant, MD, FRCP(C)

Acknowledgments

This text was reviewed by residents in the neurology training program at the Cleveland Clinic as well as at the University of Western Ontario. Their comments were crucial in re-editing this text and are much appreciated. Particular thanks to Dr. Jamie L. Steckley and Dr. Teneille Gofton of the University of Western Ontario and Dr. Guillermo Linares Tapi of the Cleveland Clinic for their cogent thoughts. Special thanks go to Dr. Lawrence Levitt, Dr. Howard Weiner, and Dr. Lorraine Spikol for reviewing and commenting on certain chapters in the book.

Contents

GLOSSARY OF COMMON NEUROLOGIC TERMS G1

Common terms used in neurology and their definitions

1. LOCALIZATION 1

The neurologic examination is designed to establish the localization of dysfunction in the nervous system. Many processes affect only specific areas in the nervous system. Thus anatomic localization becomes the foundation for diagnosis and treatment.

2. RIGHT HEMIPLEGIA 4

Right-sided weakness may be secondary to a lesion affecting the pyramidal tract anywhere from cortex to spinal cord. Evaluation of associated signs and symptoms—e.g., aphasia with cortical lesions—is made to determine the level of the lesion.

3. LEFT HEMIPLEGIA 9

Denial of illness and inattention of the left side are major features of non-dominant hemisphere dysfunction. Tests of spatial organization and attention replace aphasia testing in evaluating patients with left hemiplegia.

4. APHASIA 12

Aphasia is the major feature of dominant hemisphere dysfunction. Recognition of aphasia establishes the level of nervous system involvement, and characterization may suggest the etiology.

5. COMA 19

The clinical diagnosis of coma requires delineation of the nature and degree of central nervous system dysfunction. This chapter presents an approach to examining and evaluating the comatose patient.

Localization

There are three questions that have to be answered in assessing every patient with possible neurologic disease. These must be answered in order, or it is difficult to make an appropriate diagnosis in each case.

QUESTION 1: IS THIS A NEUROLOGIC PROBLEM?

On occasion neurologists are called to see patients with problems outside of their area of expertise. A patient with a conversion disorder who cannot move his or her leg, a patient who feels faint due to hyperventilation syndrome, and a patient who cannot walk due to malingering all have in common neurologic symptoms, but ultimately a diagnosis that is non-neurologic. None of these patients will benefit from an exhaustive neurologic evaluation, but all will benefit from appropriate supportive and therapeutic activities. Consider whether the condition is neurologic in the initial evaluation of the patient.

QUESTION 2: WHERE IN THE NERVOUS SYSTEM IS THE PROBLEM?

Where the problem is located in the nervous system is a crucial question for neurologic disorders. Without understanding where in the nervous system the problem is, one cannot understand the cause of the disorder or move forward in therapy. Lesions can either be located at a level in the nervous system (e.g., cortex, brainstem, peripheral nerve), or affect a particular neurologic system (e.g., cerebellar disorder, motor system disorder). Some diseases affect different locations in the nervous system (e.g., multiple sclerosis). Once the location of the problem is known, this guides the evaluation of the possible etiology or mechanism of the problem.

A working knowledge of basic neuroanatomy helps in localizing problems in the nervous system. Understanding the anatomy of the major ascending and descending pathways (spinothalamic tract, dorsal columns, corticospinal tract), the major cranial nerves and their brainstem connections, the visual system, and the major anatomic areas of the cortex (language areas, sensory cortex, visual cortex, motor cortex) assists in localizing lesions in the central nervous system. A working knowledge of the major root, plexus, and peripheral nerve anatomy allows effective localization of peripheral nervous system disorders.

Each level or system within the nervous system has characteristic symptoms and signs. When listening to the history or examining the patient, the examiner should consider how the signs and symptoms correlate with different nervous system locations (Table 1.1).

■ TABLE 1.1. Localization of Symptoms and Signs in the Nervous System

Location	Typical Symptoms	Typical Signs
Cortex	Cognitive, visual, language, neglect, behavior, motor, sensory, seizures, myoclonus	Field cut, aphasia, neglect, cortical sensory loss, apraxia, dementia
Brainstem	Diplopia, dysarthria, imbalance, facial weakness or numbness, weakness, altered consciousness	Combination of cranial nerve findings and long tract findings
Spinal cord	Sensory and motor symptoms below a level, bowel and bladder symptoms, stiff legs	Sensory level, motor and sensory deficits below level, reduced anal reflexes, hyperreflexia below level and upgoing toes
Nerve root	Pain down root distribution, weakness, numbness limited to root involved	Weakness, sensory loss, and reflex loss in root distribution
Plexus	Focal weakness usually in shoulder girdle or hip girdle muscles on one side, with sensory loss	Weakness of proximal muscles on one side, sensory loss in similar area not in root distribution, reflex loss
Peripheral nerve	For generalized neuropathy sensory symptoms in feet and hands, weakness, imbalance. For focal neuropathy weakness, numbness, pain in nerve distribution	"Stocking and glove" sensory loss feet + hands, decreased reflexes, distal weakness. For focal neuropathy weakness, sensory loss, reflex loss in nerve distribution
Neuromuscular junction	Fluctuating weakness, usually proximal, diplopia, dysphagia, neck weakness. No sensory symptoms or bowel and bladder symptoms	Fatigable weakness of various muscles, normal reflexes, sensory, and other neurologic examination
Muscle	Weakness, usually difficulty arising from chairs, going up stairs, combing hair	Weakness of muscles, atrophy, otherwise normal neurologic examination

■ TABLE 1.1. Localization of Symptoms and Signs
in the Nervous System (*Continued*)

System Involved	Symptoms	Signs
Motor	Weakness, spasticity, muscle twitching, dysphagia	Hyperreflexia, hyporeflexia, fasciculation, atrophy, weakness, upgoing toe
Sensory	Tingling, burning, sensory loss, unsteady gait, difficulty feeling things	Loss of pin, touch, temperature, position, vibration sensation, reflex loss
Autonomic	Blurred vision, dry mouth, loss of sweating, bowel and bladder dysfunction, postural lightheadedness	Altered pupil responses, postural hypotension, loss of R-R variability, altered gastric motility, altered sweating
Basal ganglia	Gait disorders, unusual limb movements, dysphagia, dysarthria	Parkinsonian symptoms, choreoathetosis, hemiballismus
Cerebellar	Unsteadiness, incoordination, slurred speech	Ataxic gait, nystagmus, incoordination, intention tremor, reduced reflexes

QUESTION 3: WHAT IS THE ETIOLOGY OR MECHANISM OF THE NEUROLOGIC PROBLEM?

Once the location or system is known, then the etiology can be considered. Important data from the history include the time course of the problem. Events occurring over seconds to minutes suggest stroke, migraine, seizure, hypoglycemia, or hyperventilation. Events occurring over hours to days suggest stroke, infection, rapid mass lesions, or inflammation. Events occurring over weeks to months suggest mass, chronic infection, or a degenerative process. Events occurring over years suggest a degenerative process or slow mass lesion.

Epidemiologic data from the history are very helpful. For example, octogenarians are more likely to have stroke, Alzheimer disease, and lumbar spinal stenosis than are teenagers. Patients from tropical areas are more likely to have malaria than those from Finland. Patients who have diabetes, hyperlipidemia, and hypertension are at more risk of cerebrovascular disease than those without. Patients with a family history of Huntington disease are at a well-defined risk for this autosomal-dominant disease.

Once a differential diagnosis of the etiology and mechanism is developed, a rational strategy to confirm the diagnosis can be developed. Without a stepwise analysis of each case, answering these three key questions, it is difficult to effectively treat neurologic disorders.

Right Hemiplegia

When examining a patient who has right hemiplegia (paralysis) or right hemiparesis (weakness), establish whether the lesion is cortical, subcortical, in the brainstem, or in the spinal cord (Fig. 2.1).

Hemiparesis is a sign of a corticospinal tract disorder on one side. The corticospinal tract begins in the precentral gyrus of the frontal lobes, descends through the internal capsule to the anterior brainstem, where it crosses to the opposite side in the pyramids of the medulla. It travels primarily in the lateral corticospinal tract and synapses with the lower motor neuron. A disorder in this tract is called an upper motor neuron disorder.

UPPER MOTOR NEURON FINDINGS

1. Increased reflexes.
2. Babinski sign (the toe goes up [dorsiflexes] when the lateral border of the foot is slowly stroked with a sharp point).
3. Spasticity (when the limb is passively moved there is resistance to the movement not due to contracture).
4. Clonus (e.g., when the ankle is passively dorsiflexed there is a rhythmic dorsiflexion/plantar flexion movement).

IS THE LESION CORTICAL?

1. Test the patient carefully for *aphasia* (a disorder of production or comprehension of language). Listen to spontaneous speech. Note any breakdown in fluency. Notice any errors of word or syllable choice (paraphasias). Have the patient name objects (e.g., pen, tie, watch), repeat phrases (e.g.,"no ifs, ands, or buts"), and read. Check the patient's comprehension of commands (e.g., "Touch your left thumb to your right ear. Close your eyes."). Have the patient write a sentence or two. Is the patient right-handed? **Remember, in nearly all right-handed and most left-handed people, the left hemisphere is dominant for language** (see Chapter 4).

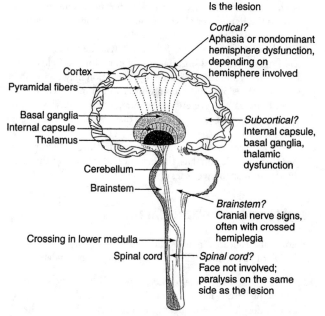

FIGURE 2.1. Establishing the level of the lesion in a patient with hemiplegia. Upper motor neurons located in the frontal and parietal cortex course down through the subcortical white matter, into the internal capsule, and through the brainstem and then cross in the lower medulla to the opposite side (decussation of the pyramids). They descend in the lateral spinal cord to synapse in the anterior horn with the lower motor neuron.

2. Check for *cortical sensory loss*. For example, test position sense, graphesthesia (write numbers on the palm), and stereognosis (have the patient identify objects placed in the hand). Touch the patient on different parts of the arm and leg, and have him or her identify where he or she is touched. Touch both sides at the same time to see if the patient notices one side only (extinction). Remember, primary sensation (pin, touch, temperature) must be intact to do such testing. **Cortical sensory loss implies a parietal or subcortical localization on the contralateral side.**

3. Are the *face and arm more affected than the leg* (suggesting lateral frontal lobe, middle cerebral artery territory in a stroke patient), or is the leg more involved (high frontal lobe or anterior cerebral artery territory)?

4. Is there *eye deviation* or a gaze preference? The eyes look toward the hemisphere involved and away from the hemiparesis in a cortical lesion (see Fig. 34.3).
5. Check carefully for a visual *field defect*. Ask the patient to identify fingers presented simultaneously in peripheral fields. *Note:* Field defects and "cortical-type" eye deviation may be found in subcortical lesions, and must be interpreted in the context of other findings. The presence of seizures, cortical sensory loss, or aphasia often will assist in accurate diagnosis, suggesting a cortical location.
6. *Are there seizures?* A hemiparesis associated with a seizure suggests a cortical lesion. Has the patient had seizures in the same distribution as the weakness?

IS THE LESION SUBCORTICAL?

Subcortical structures include the internal capsule, basal ganglia (inclusive of the globus pallidus and putamen), and thalamus.

1. Are the *face, arm, and leg equally involved* on one side (characteristic of lesions in the internal capsule)? Is there sparing of speech despite a hemiparesis, suggesting sparing of left hemisphere cortex?
2. Are there unusual movements or *dystonic postures* (seen with basal ganglia lesions)?
3. Is there a *dense sensory loss* to pin and touch in the face, arm, and leg (seen with thalamic lesions) associated with the hemiplegia (involvement of the adjacent internal capsule)? *Note:* With thalamic sensory lesions the sensory loss often splits the midline.
4. Is there visual field defect (seen with lesions of the optic tracts or optic radiations)?

IS THE LESION IN THE BRAINSTEM?

1. Look for a *crossed hemiplegia*, a classic feature of brainstem lesions. For example, a right hemiplegia from a left brainstem lesion is often accompanied by left-sided brainstem signs (e.g., left-sided dysmetria or cranial nerve palsies) at the level of the lesion.
2. Check for *ataxia*: finger-to-nose ataxia, difficulty with rapid alternating movements in the limbs, or difficulty walking heel-to-toe (tandem gait). Such ataxia may suggest a cerebellar or brainstem lesion. Remember, limb ataxia is almost always on

the same side as the lesion, so a left brainstem lesion gives left limb ataxia. Do not misinterpret weakness for ataxia.

3. Note *nystagmus*. Horizontal nystagmus is usually more marked when the patient gazes toward the side of the lesion. Vertical nystagmus is more specific for brainstem and cerebellar disease than is horizontal nystagmus.

4. Check for *hearing loss*, which occurs in the ear opposite the hemiparesis. Ask about *vertigo*, which suggests a lesion in the brainstem or cerebellum.

5. Check carefully for *sensory findings*. Characteristic findings are pain, temperature, and corneal loss on the left side of the face (involvement of descending tract of the fifth nerve) with pain and temperature loss on the right side of the body (spinothalamic tract).

6. Note *dysarthria* (slurred speech), and *dysphagia* (difficulty swallowing), which may be caused by disorders of the ninth and tenth cranial nerves (lower motor neuron), or the corticobulbar fibers supplying them (upper motor neuron). A decreased gag reflex is seen with lower motor neuron lesions. Upper motor neuron involvement causes a pseudobulbar palsy (hyperactive gag, brisk jaw jerk, and emotional lability).

7. Check for abnormal *eye movements*. In left brainstem lesions, the patient may have trouble looking to the left (gaze paresis; see Fig. 34.4), may have eye deviation to the right, or may have problems adducting the left eye (internuclear ophthalmoplegia; see Fig. 34.8).

8. In *twelfth-nerve lesions*, the tongue deviates to the side of the lesion. Thus, in a left twelfth-nerve lesion, the tongue deviates to the left as the stronger muscles on the right force the tongue left. Use the tip of the nose as a reference point. See how fast the tongue can move back and forth. Upper motor lesions slow tongue movements, leaving tongue bulk normal, whereas lower motor neuron lesions cause tongue atrophy on the affected side.

IS THE LESION IN THE SPINAL CORD?

1. The *face* is spared except for high cervical cord lesions, in which there is facial pain and temperature loss as a result of involvement of the trigeminothalamic tract, which descends one or two segments into the cervical cord.

2. Weakness is usually bilateral. If unilateral, vibration and position loss are on the same side as weakness, but pain and temperature are affected on the opposite side (Brown–Séquard syndrome; see Fig. 34.10).

■ TABLE 2.1. Tendon Reflex Grading Scale

Grade	Description
0	Absent
1+ or +	Hypoactive
2+ or ++	"Normal"
3+ or +++	Hyperactive without clonus
4+ or ++++	Hyperactive with clonus

3. A *sensory level* to pin, vibration, or sweating may be found and is most characteristic of a spinal cord lesion.
4. *Bladder and bowel* disturbances are common.
5. The sympathetic supply to the pupil descends through the cord to T1 or T2, so a Horner syndrome may occur in cervical cord lesions and high thoracic cord lesions.

Reflex testing: reflexes can be graded on a 0 to 4 scale. While this is often written as 1+, 2+, and so forth, there is no meaning to the addition of the plus sign (Table 2.1).

Suggested Readings

Brazis PW, Masdeu JC, Biller J. *Localization in Clinical Neurology.* 5th ed. Philadelphia: Lippincott Williams & Wilkins; 2007.

Gilman S, Winans-Newman S. *Manter and Gatz's Essentials of Clinical Neuroanatomy and Neurophysiology.* 7th ed. Philadelphia: Davis; 1987.

Left Hemiplegia

When examining a patient with a left hemiplegia or hemiparesis, nondominant hemisphere function rather than aphasia testing is stressed. Even in left-handed patients, the right hemisphere is usually nondominant. The remainder of cortical, subcortical, brainstem, and spinal cord testing is the same as the testing involved with right hemiplegia (see Chapter 2).

ARE THERE NONDOMINANT HEMISPHERE FINDINGS?

1. Check for inattention. Does the patient neglect the body's left side, the left side of the room, or the left side of a picture? Check for extinction by double simultaneous tactile or visual stimulation (touch both of the patient's hands at once and ask which was touched; have the patient identify fingers presented simultaneously in left and right visual fields). The right parietal cortex is important in directing attention to the left side of visual space.
2. Check for denial or "lack of concern." Does the patient say there is nothing wrong, despite having a hemiplegia, or does the patient show a lack of concern? Sometimes, a patient will identify the patient's left hand as belonging to someone else or as the examiner's hand when it is lifted into view. These are elements of anosognosia (the denial of a neurologic deficit). Such a denial is common in right parietal lesions.
3. Test for constructional apraxia. Have the patient copy a simple diagram such as a bicycle, car, or house. Have the patient draw a clock and fill in the numbers. Drawing complex figures will bring out parietal deficits missed by many other tests. The parietal lobes are key in spatial orientation, the ability to sort out spatial relationships for drawing, following a map, and performing tasks such as mental rotation.

4. Check for spatial disorientation. Does the patient get lost in the hospital, or when driving in his or her neighborhood? Lead the patient from the room. Can he or she find the way back? Can the patient figure out directions for local travel?
5. Is the patient acutely confused (reported with some nondominant hemisphere strokes)?
6. Is there a loss of the melodic and emotional content of speech or thought? Nondominant lesions may rob patients of the ability to express or understand emotional speech and make them unresponsive to usual emotional stimuli (aprosody).
7. Does the patient give up on tasks? Motor impersistence may be seen in nondominant frontal lesions. Can the tongue be held out, or an "ahhh" maintained?
8. Does the patient have difficulty dressing? Nondominant parietal lesions may cause a dressing apraxia.
9. The interlocking finger test is a simple bedside test that correlates strongly with the presence of parietal lobe dysfunction (Fig. 3.1).
10. Cortical lesions may cause focal sensory or motor changes contralateral to the area involved. The map of motor and sensory functions on the cortex is known as the homunculus (Fig. 3.2). Note that certain motor and sensory areas are more prominently represented due to their importance (hand, face areas).

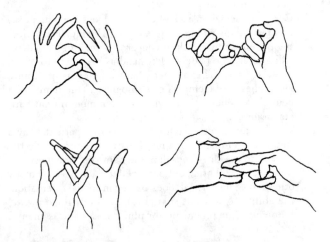

FIGURE 3.1. The interlocking finger test.

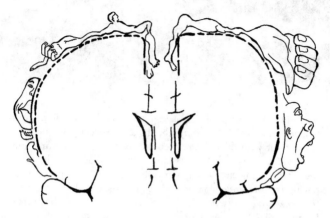

FIGURE 3.2. Sensory and motor homunculus for cortex. Coronal view, sensory on the left, motor on the right.

Suggested Readings

Critchley M. The parietal lobes. In: Denny-Brown D, Chambers RA, eds. *The Parietal Lobe and Behavior*. New York: Hafner; 1969.

Fisher CM. Left hemiplegia and motor impersistence. *J Nerv Ment Dis*. 1956;123:201.

Mesulam MM, Waxman S, Geschwind N, et al. Acute confusional states with right middle cerebral artery infarctions. *J Neurol Neurosurg Psychiatry*. 1976;39:84.

Moo, LR, Slotnick SD, Tesoro MA, et al. Interlocking finger test: a bedside screen for parietal lobe dysfunction. *JNNP*. 2003;74:530–532.

Aphasia

Aphasia is a disorder of language. The patient with aphasia uses language incorrectly, or comprehends it imperfectly. In contrast, the patient with dysarthria articulates poorly, but grammar and word choice are correct. Aphasia may show up as difficulty finding words, using the wrong words, having trouble repeating, or having trouble understanding what others say. Aphasia must be recognized clinically because it localizes the lesion to the cortex (or immediately under the cortex), and usually to the left hemisphere. There are three exceptions:

1. Some (fewer than 50%) left-handed people use the right hemisphere for speech.
2. Anomic aphasias, in which the inability to generate word names is the predominant feature, may result from metabolic disorders or space-occupying lesions with pressure effects.
3. Basal ganglia and thalamic lesions, especially in the left hemisphere, may produce aphasia.

Because different types of aphasia may imply different localizations, the clinician first must recognize that aphasia exists and then characterize it.

ANATOMY OF APHASIA

Language "ability" is a function of the left hemisphere for almost all right-handed and for most left-handed individuals. The "language areas" are located in the distribution of the middle cerebral artery surrounding the sylvian fissure (frontal and temporal cortex). Important areas for speech include the Broca area of the inferior frontal lobe, the Wernicke area in the superior temporal lobe, the arcuate fasciculus, the supramarginal gyrus, and the nearby cortex (Fig. 4.1).

The Broca and Wernicke areas are connected by the arcuate fasciculus. The *Wernicke area* lies next to the primary auditory cortex, involves the "understanding" of auditory input as language, and monitors speech output. It is connected with the

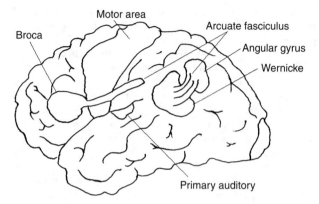

FIGURE 4.1. Important areas involved in language function.

supramarginal gyrus, a center for integrating sensory and other association information.

The arcuate fasciculus is a white-matter tract leading to the *Broca area*, which in turn, is responsible for the motor part or "production" of language. The Broca area helps translate the information carried from other language areas into phonation and speech output.

TYPES OF APHASIA

Although there is a continuum of aphasia and its severity, patients with aphasia can be subcategorized depending on the type of problem they have. These subcategories have anatomic and pathologic significance.

Broca Aphasia

With Broca aphasia, the lesion is in or near the Broca area (inferior frontal cortex near the motor strip). Speech is *nonfluent* (halting), produced with great effort, and poorly articulated. There is marked reduction in total speech, which may be "telegraphic" with the omission of articles (the, an) or word endings. *Comprehension* of written and verbal speech is good, except where grammar is required. For example, a patient may have difficulty with a question such as, "If a tiger is eaten by a lion, which one is still alive?" *Repetition* of single words may be good, although it is done with great effort. Phrase repetition is poor, especially phrases containing words such as "if," "and," or "but." The patient always *writes* in an aphasic manner, and writing is affected even in a subtle aphasia. *Object naming* is usually poor, although it may be better than spontaneous speech. *Hemiparesis* (usually greater in the face and arm than the leg) is present in larger lesions because the motor cortex is close to the Broca area. The patient is *aware* of this deficit, but is frustrated and frequently depressed. Interestingly, the patient may be able to *hum a melody* normally. However, a musician may have deficits in producing music. Curses or other ejaculatory speech may be well articulated. These exceptions are the result of right-hemisphere mechanisms for such emotional speech. Buccolingual apraxia, which is difficulty producing facial movements to command, not caused by poor comprehension or paralysis, may be present. It is demonstrated by having the patient try to protrude the tongue, blow out the cheeks, or whistle.

Wernicke Aphasia

With Wernicke aphasia, the lesion is in or near the Wernicke area of the dominant temporal lobe. *Speech is fluent* with normal rhythm and articulation, but it conveys information poorly, because of meandering, indirect phrases (circumlocutions), use of nonsense words (neologisms), and incorrect words (paraphasic errors). The patient uses wrong words and sounds. For example: "letter" for "ladder" (phonemic paraphasia), or "orange" for "apple" (semantic paraphasia). The patient is unable to *comprehend* written or verbal speech. The content of *writing* is abnormal, as is speech, although the penmanship may be good. *Repetition* is poor. *Object naming* is poor. *Hemiparesis* is mild or absent, because the lesion is far from the motor cortex. A hemianopsia or quadrantanopsia may be present owing to involvement of optic radiations passing through the affected temporal lobe. Patients do not realize the nature of their deficit, and usually are not depressed in the acute stage. They may exhibit elements of paranoia for this reason. This type of aphasia is commonly the result of an embolic event to the superior temporal gyrus.

Conduction Aphasia

Conduction aphasia is caused by a lesion in the posterior part of the superior temporal gyrus or supramarginal gyrus. It functionally disconnects the anterior and posterior speech areas. *Speech* is fluent, but conveys information imperfectly. Paraphasic errors are common. The patient can *comprehend* spoken or written phrases containing small grammatical words. *Repetition* is the most severely affected, especially for phrases containing grammatical words and nonsense syllables. There is difficulty *naming objects*. *Written language* is impaired, although penmanship is preserved. *Hemiparesis*, if present, is mild.

Anomic Aphasia

Anomic aphasia is the least localizing of the aphasias, and may be seen with a variety of disorders of the dominant hemisphere. It is a common manifestation of Alzheimer disease. It may be seen as patients recover from a more severe form of aphasia as a residual deficit. *Speech* is fluent but conveys information poorly, because of paraphasic errors and circumlocutions. (Literally, patients talk around words they cannot recall.) The main problem is naming. This can be demonstrated by having the patient name as many animals as possible in 1 minute. A person should be able to name 10 or more. The patient can *understand* written and spoken speech. There is no *hemiplegia*. *Comprehension* and *repetition* are normal, although these may be difficult to assess in a patient who is confused (e.g., in metabolic encephalopathy).

Global Aphasia

Global aphasia is seen with large lesions affecting both the Wernicke and Broca areas. Marked hemiparesis occurs, in addition to inability to comprehend and to speak. Global aphasia is seen with large infarcts in the middle cerebral artery territory, and often is caused by occlusion of the left internal carotid artery or trunk of the middle cerebral artery.

Other Aphasic Syndromes

Aphasias may occur because of lesions located outside the peri-sylvian region, in "border zone" areas. **These "transcortical aphasias" are characterized by a relative sparing of repetition, despite other language difficulties.** The clinical importance of transcortical aphasias is that they typically are related to pro-longed hypotension, or hypoxia (e.g., after cardiac arrest). These patients often repeat and read well, but have diminished fluency (anterior border zone lesions), or comprehend poorly (posterior border zone lesions).

EXAMINATION OF THE PATIENT WITH APHASIA

First, establish whether the patient is aphasic, and then determine the nature of the aphasia. Remember, it may be difficult to determine whether a patient who is inattentive or confused is aphasic.

1. *Listen to speech output.* Is it fluent or nonfluent? If fluent, the lesion is posterior; if nonfluent, it usually is anterior.
2. Can the patient *read and write* without errors? If so, aphasia is not present.
3. Check *naming.* In the patient with aphasia, naming almost always is impaired.
4. Check for *repetition.* If the patient is aphasic but can repeat, there is a transcortical aphasia.
5. Can the patient comprehend simple yes or no questions? Comprehension is relatively spared in Broca aphasia.
6. Is there *hemiparesis?* If so, the lesion is anterior, involving the motor area.
7. To delineate the various types of fluent aphasias, check whether the patient is fluent, can comprehend, and can repeat (Table 4.1).

THE IMPORTANCE OF DEFINING THE APHASIA

The definition of aphasia localizes the *level* of the nervous system lesion. If aphasia is present, the lesion is usually in the left cerebral cortex. Someone with difficulty using the right hand and a mild aphasia has hemisphere disease, not a brachial plexus lesion.

Aphasia on a vascular basis implies dysfunction of middle cerebral artery territory and often is caused by disease of the internal

■ TABLE 4.1. Taxonomic Classification of Aphasia

Type of Aphasia	Is Patient Fluent?	Does Patient Comprehend?	Can Patient Repeat?
Broca	No	Yes	No
Wernicke	Yes	No	No
Conduction	Yes	Yes	No
Anomic	Yes	Yes	Yes
Transcortical motor	No	Yes	Yes
Transcortical sensory	Yes	No	Yes
Transcortical mixed (isolation)	No	No	Yes
Global	No	No	No

carotid in the neck. Marked stenosis of the internal carotid may be surgically correctable, and if recognized and treated in time, a mild or transient aphasia may be prevented from becoming global.

The sudden onset of fluent aphasia without hemiparesis often means an embolus to the posterior branch of the middle cerebral artery. Look for an embolic focus in the heart, or in the carotid artery. If the heart is the source, anticoagulation should be considered; if the carotid is the suspected source, angiography usually is performed in search of a surgically remediable lesion. Remember the clinical rule: the sudden onset of aphasia without hemiparesis suggests embolus.

PROGNOSIS

The prognosis of aphasia in a given patient depends on the location and extent of the lesion, as well as the underlying pathology. Patients with global aphasia have a poor prognosis and almost never recover completely. Patients with anomic, conduction, and transcortical aphasias have a good prognosis, and complete recovery occurs frequently. Patients with Broca and Wernicke aphasia have an intermediate prognosis and show a wide range of outcomes. In general, patients with traumatic cases of aphasia do better than those in whom stroke is the cause. Newer techniques of imaging, particularly diffusion-perfusion magnetic resonance imaging, have revealed that many aphasias associated with subcortical infarctions likely result from cortical hypoperfusion, and may be reversible with restored perfusion. The bulk of evidence indicates that speech therapy improves the outcome in aphasia. New treatment techniques, such as comprehension treatment programs and visual communication therapy, are being used to help the patient with aphasia. A team approach to rehabilitation with close cooperation between the neurologist, speech pathologist, and psychologist benefits the patient greatly.

RELATED DISORDERS

1. *Apraxia* is a disturbance of purposeful movement that cannot be accounted for by elementary motor or sensory impairments, and by impaired comprehension or cooperation. For example, in dressing apraxia, the patient is unable to dress despite adequate motor power. Apraxias occur commonly in association with aphasic syndromes, and usually involve the "disconnection" of one brain area from another.

2. *Agnosias* are disorders of recognition that are not accounted for by elementary perceptual disturbances. For example, visual agnosia is a disorder of recognition not accounted for by a primary disorder of vision. In this condition, the person can see an object but cannot identify it visually. Once the person holds it in the hand, he or she usually can identify it by touch.

3. *Gerstmann syndrome* refers to a lesion of the left angular gyrus that causes difficulty writing (agraphia), left–right confusion, difficulty identifying fingers (finger agnosia), and difficulty with calculations (acalculia).

DISCONNECTION SYNDROMES

Disconnection syndromes occur when one part of the cortex is disconnected from the other. Examples include the following:

1. *Alexia without agraphia.* The patient can write but cannot read: lesion in the left occipital region and adjacent corpus callosum. In this syndrome, the preserved right occipital lobe is disconnected from the left-hemisphere language areas.

2. *Balint syndrome.* The patient has visual inattention, and cannot direct gaze to specific points in the visual field despite full extraocular movement (optic ataxia and visual apraxia): bilateral parieto-occipital lesions.

3. *Pure word deafness.* The patient cannot interpret words or repeat what is said, but can hear sounds and interpret written language: deep left temporal lobe lesion or bilateral temporal lobe lesions in the primary auditory cortex.

4. *Ideomotor apraxia.* The patient uses left hand well for all functions, except those suggested by verbal commands: lesions in left frontal cortex and adjacent corpus callosum.

Suggested Readings

Albert ML. Treatment of aphasia. *Arch Neurol.* 1998;55:1417–1419.

Damasio AR. Aphasia. *N Engl J Med.* 1992;326:531–539.

Jordan LC, Hillis AE. Disorders of speech and language: aphasia, apraxia and dysarthria. *Curr Opin Neurol.* 2006;19:580–585.

Moreaud O. Balint syndrome. *Arch Neurol.* 2003;60:1329–1331.

Saffran EM. Aphasia and the relationship of language and brain. *Semin Neurol.* 2000;20:409–418.

Coma

Proper evaluation of the comatose patient involves obtaining a history from family and friends, performing a rapid directed physical and neurologic examination, and obtaining certain laboratory studies, while the patient's airway and vital signs are protected. These tasks often are done simultaneously (e.g., one member of the medical team secures the airway, while another talks to the family). An attempt is made to delineate the cause of coma in hopes of finding a treatable process. Treatable causes of coma include metabolic derangements, ingestions, and at times, supratentorial processes in the brain (e.g., epidural hematoma). Anatomically, coma implies bilateral hemisphere dysfunction; structural, drug-induced, or metabolic, unilateral hemisphere disease with compression of the brainstem (e.g., epidural hematoma); or brainstem dysfunction (e.g., pontine hemorrhage or compression from a posterior fossa mass). If certain basic points are established when examining the comatose patient, the extent of structural central nervous system (CNS) derangement and the cause usually can be determined. One must determine if the patient is comatose or in another state of altered responsiveness (Table 5.1). Comatose patients do not awaken to stimulation of any kind. They may respond with vocalizations, movements, and changes in blood pressure or pulse, but do not interact in any meaningful way with the examiner.

ABCs

Before obtaining a history and physical, make sure the patient's *a*irway, *b*reathing, and *c*irculation (ABCs) are stable. Draw blood for glucose, and give 1/2 to 1 amp of 50% dextrose intravenously (IV) (for hypoglycemia). Give thiamine 100 mg IV to avoid precipitating Wernicke syndrome in patients with alcoholism. Although traditionally it was considered risky to give glucose before providing thiamine, there are no data to support this supposition. Consider naloxone for narcotic ingestion. Then, proceed with history, physical, and other diagnostic testing. **Hypoglycemia is a common and treatable cause of coma.**

■ **TABLE 5.1. States of Decreased Responsiveness**

Unresponsive but Appears Awake
    Drowsiness—reduced alertness
    Abulic state—frontal lobe disease
    Psychiatric diseases—e.g., catatonia
    Locked-in syndromes—e.g., pontine infarction
    Nonconvulsive status epilepticus
Decreased Responsiveness and Appears Asleep
    Stupor—awakens when stimulated but returns to unresponsiveness
    Coma—no awakening to stimulation
    Psychogenic unresponsiveness

HISTORY

1. Learn from family or friends whether the patient has a preexisting condition that may explain the coma. Does the patient have diabetes? Is he or she a drug addict or an alcoholic? Does the patient take sleeping pills? Has the patient been depressed? Has the patient sustained recent head trauma? Were there episodes of a similar nature in the past?
2. If a preexisting medical condition exists, is there a factor that may have exacerbated it, and precipitated the coma (e.g., chronic liver disease, gastrointestinal bleeding, uremia and infection, a seizure disorder, or failure to take anticonvulsant medication)?
3. A review of all medications, including sleeping pills, and all medical conditions may give hints about the cause of coma.
4. Review the events leading up to the coma. A prodromal febrile illness may suggest meningitis or encephalitis, whereas a despondent patient may suggest the possibility of an overdose.

EXAMINATION

Observe the patient carefully:

1. Is there *decorticate posturing* (arm flexion with leg extension); implying hemisphere or diencephalon dysfunction that may be caused by destructive lesions, or may be secondary to a metabolic derangement?
2. Is there *decerebrate posturing* (extension of legs and arms), implying dysfunction of midbrain or upper pons on a structural or metabolic basis?

3. Is the patient yawning, swallowing, or licking the lips? If so, coma cannot be deep and brainstem function is probably intact.
4. Are there repetitive, multifocal, myoclonic jerks (brief muscle twitches in varied muscle groups)? These are characteristic of metabolic encephalopathies, such as hypoxia or uremia. Profound multifocal myoclonus may occur after anoxic injury and implies a poor prognosis.
5. Is there evidence of seizure activity, which sometimes may be as subtle as eye blinking, eye deviation, or facial myoclonus? If so, consider antiepileptic drugs and electroencephalogram (EEG) monitoring. Continued nonconvulsive status may cause irreversible brain injury if not treated.
6. Does the patient move only one side, suggesting a hemiparesis?
7. Are there needle track marks, signs of chronic liver disease, or signs of trauma? Is there a stiff neck, suggesting meningitis? Is the patient poorly groomed and ill appearing, suggesting the possibility of Wernicke disease?

WHAT IS THE RESPIRATORY PATTERN?

Cheyne–Stokes respiration (a crescendo–decrescendo breathing pattern with apneic pauses in-between) implies bilateral hemisphere dysfunction with an intact brainstem. It often accompanies metabolic disorders and congestive heart failure. Rarely, it may be the first sign of transtentorial herniation.

Central neurogenic hyperventilation (rapid deep breathing), usually indicates damage to the brainstem tegmentum between midbrain and pons.

Apneustic breathing consists of a prolonged inspiratory phase followed by an expiratory pause, and usually is seen in pontine infarction.

Ataxic (irregular or agonal) breathing is usually a preterminal event signifying disruption of medullary centers.

Remember, significant damage to the brainstem rarely is accompanied by a normal breathing pattern. *Coma with hyperventilation frequently signifies a metabolic derangement:*

• Metabolic acidosis: diabetes, uremia, lactic acidosis, poisoning.
• Respiratory alkalosis: salicylates, hepatic failure.

Coma with hypoventilation frequently implies generalized CNS depression secondary to a drug overdose, and also occurs in patients with chronic pulmonary disease and CO_2 retention.

DOES THE PATIENT RESPOND TO EXTERNAL STIMULI?

1. Apply a noxious stimulus to determine whether the patient is unresponsive. Noxious stimuli may elicit decorticate or decerebrate posturing, and thus give a clue to the level of brain damage or dysfunction. Movement of only one side is crucial evidence of a hemiparesis caused by brainstem or supratentorial disease. Withdrawal implies purposeful or voluntary behavior.
2. Test for a voluntary response. Are there inconsistencies in the depth of coma? Does the patient avoid noxious stimuli in a directed fashion? Let the patient's hand fall toward the face and see if the patient resists (a check for malingering).
3. Tickling the nose with a cotton swab is a strong noxious stimulus. See if the patient grimaces, opens the eyes, or withdraws the head.
4. Check for a response of the limbs to pain. Is there a low-level reflex, such as flexion, extension, or adduction? Abduction of shoulder or hip usually indicates a higher level (cortical) response.

EXAMINE THE PUPILS CAREFULLY

Note the size, equality, and light reaction of the pupils:

1. A comatose patient with metabolic intoxication may have no response to external stimuli, absent doll's eyes, and corneal reflexes, and yet have intact pupillary responses. Such cases are often secondary to barbiturate ingestion. Remember, reactive pupils in a comatose patient without other responses suggest a metabolic cause.
2. Normal-sized, reactive pupils imply an intact midbrain. Midbrain damage usually produces dilated pupils that do not react to light but may fluctuate in size.
3. Atropine or scopolamine poisoning causes large unreactive pupils that give the false impression of a structural lesion.
4. Pontine damage produces pinpoint pupils that react to bright light when viewed with a magnifying glass. Heroin and pilocarpine also produce pinpoint pupils.
5. A unilaterally fixed, dilated pupil is seen with damage to the third nerve and often is a valuable early sign of a mass effect from a laterally placed supratentorial lesion (see Chapter 31). It also may be caused by direct damage to the midbrain, such as by a stroke in the basilar artery territory.

CHECK CORNEAL REFLEXES AND THE DOLL'S EYE MANEUVER

Absence of corneal reflexes and the doll's eye sign usually means pontine damage or dysfunction. Make sure there is no cervical spine fracture before performing the doll's eye maneuver. Turn the head from side to side to see if the eyes conjugately deviate to the side opposite that to which the head is turned. This may be done in a vertical direction as well. Altered horizontal eye movements usually indicate a pontine lesion, whereas altered vertical eye movements often indicate a midbrain lesion.

If there is no doll's eye response, use ice water irrigation (100–200 mL in each ear), a strong stimulus of the oculovestibular reflex pathway. Be sure that there is no wax in the ears and that the tympanic membranes are intact; check one ear at a time. Tonically deviated eyes to the side of the irrigation (a "normal" brainstem response in a comatose patient) signify that some brainstem function is intact. Absence of the oculovestibular response implies severe depression of brainstem function because it involves a large amount of brainstem territory: cranial nerves III, IV, and VI; the medial longitudinal fasciculus; and the vestibular apparatus.

MOTOR SYSTEM EXAMINATION

Hyperreflexia, and *upgoing* toes or hemiplegia, usually mean a structural CNS lesion is the cause of coma. Some exceptions include hepatic coma, hypoglycemia, and uremia, which may be associated with focal signs or hyperreflexia. Nonetheless, these exceptions should be diagnosed quickly by laboratory studies.

OTHER PHYSICAL FINDINGS

Careful physical examination may detect other clues to the cause of coma (e.g., signs of head trauma in epidural hematoma, barrel chest in pulmonary failure, hepatomegaly in hepatic coma, feeble pulse and hypotension in cardiogenic shock, and stiff neck in meningitis or subarachnoid hemorrhage). There may be cyanosis with hypoxia, or "cherry red" appearance in carbon monoxide poisoning. Hypothermia may be associated with barbiturate or ethanol ingestion, whereas hyperthermia may occur in heat stroke.

LABORATORY STUDIES

Laboratory studies must be carried out to exclude metabolic causes of coma, such as hypoglycemia, hypercapnia, hypercalcemia, uremia, hepatic failure, electrolyte disturbance, or toxin ingestion. When clinically appropriate, a computed tomography scan is indicated to rule out intracranial hemorrhage (subdural, epidural, or intracerebral), abscess, tumor, or hydrocephalus. An EEG is helpful if seizures are suspected; it is also useful for metabolic encephalopathy (slowing and triphasic waves), or for psychogenic coma (normal EEG). A lumbar puncture may be needed to detect infection or subarachnoid hemorrhage; although one must be certain that there is no shift of midline structures before the lumbar puncture. Other therapeutic measures, such as treatment of increased intracranial pressure or gastric lavage after ingestions, may be required. Remember, for a patient with coma, the neurologic examination should define whether a diffuse disorder, structural supratentorial disease, or infratentorial disease is most likely. The history and general examination provide clues to the etiology of coma.

DETERMINING BRAIN DEATH IN ADULTS

With the advent of long-term ventilation, as well as the development of organ transplantation in the 1960s, there was a need to define when irreversible cessation of brain function had occurred. This irreversible cessation of brain function is known as brain death, or death by brain criteria. A 1995 American Academy of Neurology expert panel developed guidelines for determining brain death in adults, which have been reaffirmed in subsequent reviews (see reference). Key points in determining brain death in adults include:

1. The proximate cause of the brain death is known, and known to be irreversible.
2. Confounding factors such as core temperature below 90°F, drug intoxication, severe metabolic and acid–base disorder are ruled out.
3. There is an absence of brainstem reflexes (no pupil response, no oculocephalic reflex or cold water caloric response, no corneal reflex, no jaw reflex or no gag reflex).
4. Apnea testing as described in the guideline shows no respiratory movements with an appropriate rise in PCO_2.
5. Pitfalls in the diagnosis include severe facial trauma, prior pupil abnormalities, toxic levels of a variety of medications, or

CO_2 retention. Occasionally, patients with severe acute peripheral neuropathies may appear to be "brain dead," with normal EEG activity but an inability to move.

6. Certain clinical phenomena can be seen in patients who otherwise meet brain death criteria, and probably reflect spinal cord function: spontaneous limb movements other than pathological flexion or extension; respiratory-like movements without tidal volume change; sweating, blushing, and tachycardia; deep tendon reflexes; and Babinski response.

7. Confirmatory testing is optional in determining brain death, which remains a clinical diagnosis. A repeated exam 6 hours after initial exam is recommended. One or more of the following tests can be used as a confirmatory test:

Conventional angiography.
EEG.
TCD.
Technicium-99m hexamethylprophyleneamineoxime brain scan.
Somatosensory evoked potentials.

All have technical limitations that should be known to the physician using these tests.

Brain death should be determined by a physician skilled in this difficult area, who is aware of the criteria, pitfalls, and possible confirmatory testing for this entity.

Suggested Readings

Giacino JT, Ashwal S, Childs N, et al. The minimally conscious state: definition and diagnostic criteria. *Neurology*. 2002;58:349–353.

Hamel MB, Phillips R, Teno J, et al. Cost effectiveness of aggressive care for patients with non-traumatic coma. *Crit Care Med*. 2002;30:1191–1196.

Hypothermia after cardiac arrest study group. Mild therapeutic hypothermia to improve the neurologic outcome after cardiac arrest. *N Engl J Med*. 2002;346:549–556.

Stevens RD, Nyquist PA. Coma, delirium, and cognitive dysfunction in critical illness. *Crit Care Clin*. 2006;22:787–804.

Wijdicks EFM. The diagnosis of brain death. *N Engl J Med*. 2001;344:1215.

Young BG. Evoked-response testing for prognosis in anoxic-ischemic encephalopathy: a cool approach. *Crit Care Med*. 2005;33:1868–1869.

6

Vertigo-Dizziness

William Osler once was quoted as saying that no physician can hear the presenting complaint of "dizziness" without experiencing a sinking feeling. Although dizziness as a presentation is one of the most common in medicine, most physicians are uncomfortable with the diagnosis of this complaint.

The analysis of dizziness starts with having the patient define what he or she means by dizziness. **Ask the patient to define his or her dizziness.**

Dizziness is a nonspecific description of a variety of bodily sensations. Most patients, when asked, can describe their sensations more specifically and usefully. Do not allow the patient to get away with just saying "dizziness."

1. Vertigo: a sense of spinning of self, or the environment. Vertigo indicates a vestibular system disorder.
2. Light-headedness: a feeling of faintness, or that one might pass out. This is associated with reduced perfusion to the brain from a variety of causes.
3. Unsteadiness: a feeling that one cannot stand or walk reliably. Unsteadiness may be caused by a variety of neurologic problems.
4. Wooziness: a less well-defined feeling of being "not right" or "unwell," sometimes indicating anxiety.

ASSESSING VERTIGO

Vertigo implies a problem in the vestibular system. A disorder in the ear, eighth nerve, brainstem, or temporal lobe (the vestibular system) can cause vertigo. Occasionally, cervical disorders can cause vertigo by alteration of afferent sensory flow from receptors in the neck muscles (cervicogenic vertigo).

An important task is to decide whether the cause is *peripheral* (labyrinth, vestibular, or cochlear nerve) or *central* (brainstem, cerebellum, or cerebral cortex).

History of Vertigo

Questions to ask:

1. Does the vertigo last seconds, and is it related to a change in head position? (Positional vertigo).
2. Is there associated nausea, vomiting, or headache? (These may be seen with migraine or intracranial processes.)
3. Are symptoms of diplopia, dysarthria, focal weakness, or numbness present? (These suggest a brainstem lesion.)
4. Is there tinnitus or deafness? (These suggest eighth nerve or ear involvement.)
5. Is the patient taking many medications? (Medications may cause vertigo.).

Examination of the Vertiginous Patient

1. Specifically check the ear canal and hearing (listening to a watch tick, the spoken voice, and finger-rubbing screens three basic frequencies).
2. Perform a complete neurologic examination with special attention to cranial nerves, coordination, and the presence of nystagmus (horizontal, vertical, or rotatory).
3. Check for positional vertigo and nystagmus by having the patient go from a sitting to a supine position, while quickly turning the head to the side and with the neck extended 30 degrees. Note nystagmus, latency of the response, associated vertigo, and fatigability of the response.
4. Caloric testing (minimal ice water caloric test) may be performed. Patient lies supine with the head elevated 30 degrees. Irrigate each ear with 0.2 mL ice water (tuberculin syringe). Notice any asymmetry between the response in each ear.

Is the Vertigo Peripheral or Central in Origin?

With vertigo, a major goal of the clinician is to decide whether the lesion is peripheral (labyrinth, vestibular, or cochlear nerve) or central (brainstem, cerebellum, or cerebral cortex). A careful history is often helpful in making this distinction.

Peripheral lesions causing vertigo may be associated with deafness and tinnitus (signs of eighth-nerve dysfunction); there are no central signs. If caloric testing reproduces the patient's dizziness or there is a unilaterally decreased caloric response, the lesion is usually peripheral. Central lesions are defined by central nervous system (CNS) signs or symptoms (e.g., ataxia, cranial nerve abnormalities, diplopia, dysarthria, papilledema). In peripheral vestibulopathy, the patient falls toward the side of the lesion and away from the fast component of nystagmus. In central lesions such as cerebellar infarction, the patient falls toward the side of the lesion and toward the fast component of nystagmus. *Vertical nystagmus* is a sign of brainstem disease unless the patient is taking medication (especially barbiturates). *Rotary or torsional nystagmus* generally is seen with peripheral lesions.

Testing for Positional Nystagmus

Testing for positional nystagmus may be helpful in discriminating peripheral from central vertigo. The Dix–Hallpike maneuver is used. The patient is taken from a sitting position to lying flat with the head extended over the edge of the bed 30 degrees, with the head turned to the left or the right. Positional nystagmus of peripheral origin usually begins 3 to 10 seconds after assuming the new head position (latency of the response), is commonly associated with vertigo and nausea, lasts up to 10 seconds, and is fatigable (it becomes harder to elicit the nystagmus after several consecutive tries) (Table 6.1). *Positional nystagmus of central origin* begins immediately, may last longer than 10 seconds, and is not fatigable; nausea and vertigo are not prominent. Rarer forms of *benign paroxysmal positional vertigo* (BPPV) are highlighted in the appendix to this chapter.

Is the Lesion Peripheral?

Middle ear disease may affect the labyrinth. Check for otitis or a history of recent ear infection, and other abnormalities of the tympanic membrane. Establish whether the patient has been exposed to ototoxic drugs.

Ménière disease is a recurrent disease with a characteristic triad: episodic vertigo, tinnitus, and deafness. The underlying mechanism probably relates to swelling of the endolymphatic space. Before vertigo appears, there may be a buildup with tinnitus and "stuffiness"; the attack is violent and includes nausea, vomiting,

■ **TABLE 6.1. Differentiation of Peripheral Versus Central Positional Nystagmus**

	Peripheral	Central
Latency	3–10 seconds	None
Fatigability	Yes	No
Associated symptoms	Nausea, vomiting	Diplopia, dysarthria
Vertical nystagmus	Absent	May be present
Rotatory nystagmus	Common	Uncommon

sweating, and decreased hearing. Patients often note a "full" feeling on the side of the affected ear. Nystagmus is present only during the attack, and the direction may vary. Ménière disease occurs in patients from the ages of 30 to 60 years, and is accompanied by residual tinnitus and hearing loss after multiple attacks. The vertigo is sudden, recurrent, and severe; it usually lasts 1 to 2 hours. Treatment includes bed rest, sedatives, fluids, antihistamines, and antiemetics during the attack. Prophylactically, some physicians use diuretics and sodium restriction. A recent Cochrane review of diuretic therapy found no good evidence supporting diuretic therapy in this syndrome. Surgical therapy (endolymphatic shunt) is recommended in some chronic cases.

BPPV occurs when the patient turns the head or changes position; it can be reproduced by testing for positional nystagmus. There is no hearing loss, calorics are normal, and the disorder may be self-limited. In patients with BPPV, a variety of exercises may terminate the symptoms by moving otolithic particles away from the affected portion of the inner ear, where they are altering movements of the labyrinthine hair cells (Brandt–Daroff exercises, modified Epley maneuver). In some cases, more prolonged bouts of vertigo may be helped by these maneuvers.

Acute labyrinthitis may be secondary to bacterial or viral infections. The onset may be sudden, with severe vertigo and gastrointestinal symptoms. The attack lasts 1 to 3 days. There usually is spontaneous nystagmus toward the good ear, hearing may or may not be affected, and calorics are usually normal. Treatment is symptomatic (i.e., bed rest plus meclizine or lorazepam).

Vestibular neuronitis refers to sudden attacks of vertigo and nausea with no auditory signs or symptoms. Caloric testing shows hypofunction of the affected side, which serves to distinguish it from labyrinthitis. Treatment is symptomatic.

Posttraumatic vertigo is common, and damage to the labyrinth is the postulated mechanism because symptoms are those of peripheral vestibulopathy. The prognosis is good, with symptoms subsiding over a period of weeks.

Does the Lesion Begin Peripherally and Then Spread Centrally?

Acoustic neuroma begins from sheath cells of the vestibular portion of the eighth nerve in the internal auditory canal; thus tinnitus, decreased hearing (e.g., trouble hearing on the phone), and dizziness or disequilibrium are early complaints. As the tumor grows into the cerebellopontine angle, cranial nerve dysfunction (loss of corneal reflex, facial weakness) and cerebellar signs become prominent.

Because such tumors can be small and confined to the internal auditory canal, a contrast-enhanced magnetic resonance imaging (MRI) is the imaging modality of choice. Brainstem auditory evoked response is a sensitive screening tool for acoustic neuroma.

Is the Lesion Central?

Posterior fossa tumors may cause vertigo or dizziness; look for cerebellar and other brainstem signs. Check for evidence of increased intracranial pressure in patients with vertigo and headache by examination of the fundi.

Vascular disease (vertebrobasilar insufficiency) may cause vertigo. To establish that vertebrobasilar insufficiency is the cause, note other brainstem symptoms (diplopia, slurred speech, numbness, or trouble swallowing) or signs (cranial nerve dysfunction, motor or sensory loss). Other important points include the following:

1. Dizziness or vertigo alone may be the *first* sign of vertebrobasilar insufficiency, but most patients have accompanying signs or symptoms of brainstem dysfunction.
2. The *lateral medullary syndrome* (Chapter 16) may begin with vertigo.
3. *Cerebellar hemorrhage or infarction* may begin with the acute onset of dizziness, vomiting, inability to walk or stand, and severe headache (see Chapter 16).
4. If dizziness is accompanied by *eighth-nerve dysfunction* only, it is probably not vascular in origin.
5. Vertigo is seldom a feature of carotid artery disease.

Temporal lobe epilepsy is an important though rare cause of dizziness and vertigo. Note a history of staring spells, automatisms, déjà vu, or abdominal pain. Workup for this seizure disorder should include a sleep electroencephalogram. Effective treatment is available (antiepileptic drugs).

Basilar migraine may be associated with vertigo, and is characterized by symptoms in the basilar artery territory. Check for vertigo, visual disturbances (including scotomata), tinnitus, blackouts, and associated complaints of throbbing occipital headache. It usually occurs in young females. Treatment includes prophylactic migraine medication. Patients with migraine have a higher frequency of vertigo or dizziness than the general population. **Migraine is a common cause of hard-to-diagnose vertigo and nausea.**

Dizziness after *head trauma* may be the result of eighth-nerve injury, benign paroxysmal vertigo, or represent posttraumatic epilepsy.

Multiple sclerosis may present with dizziness or *diplopia* as a result of brainstem involvement (see Chapter 21).

Occasionally patients with acute cervical spine disease may develop vertigo due to stimulation of cervical afferents to the vestibular system.

Laboratory Evaluation of Vertigo

Laboratory studies that may prove useful in the evaluation of the patient with vertigo include the following:

1. Brainstem auditory evoked responses; particularly sensitive for acoustic neuromas.
2. Electronystagmography; particularly sensitive for peripheral labyrinthopathies.
3. MRI for structural lesions of the posterior fossa, eighth nerve, and cochlea.

The history and physical examination are more important than laboratory testing in patients with "dizziness."

Treatment of Vertigo

BPPV is treated with either the modified Epley maneuver or the Brandt–Daroff exercises, and most patients benefit from these maneuvers (Fig. 6.1).

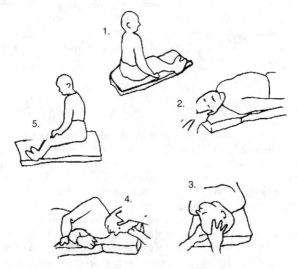

FIGURE 6.1. Modified Epley maneuver.

Drugs that may be useful in the treatment of vertigo include meclizine, other antihistamines, diazepam or lorazepam, and anticholinergics. The patient also should be advised to avoid sudden positional changes. Limiting intake of caffeine, nicotine, alcohol, and salt may be of benefit. In some cases of severe incapacitating vertigo, surgery (such as closure of an endolymphatic fistula) is necessary. A graded series of exercises may be helpful in other patients with chronic vertigo of peripheral or central origin. Antiepileptic drugs are useful in the rare patient who has vertigo as a manifestation of simple partial seizures.

LIGHT-HEADEDNESS

A common cause of "dizziness" is actually light-headedness. Most patients, when asked, tell the examiner that they feel like they are going to pass out. Another way to ask the question is to see if they have ever fainted, and then ask if this feels like the symptoms they had with fainting. When the symptom of light-headedness is established, a search for causes of low blood pressure should be undertaken. Blood pressure lying and standing should be checked. Assessment for cardiac risk factors and sources of arrhythmia may be important. Medications or diseases causing postural hypotension should be considered. In young people with light-headedness and syncope, neurocardiogenic syncope is common and diagnosed using a prolonged tilt table test. Disorders of cardiac output may also cause these symptoms. Finally, migraine is commonly associated with light-headedness and even syncope due to autonomic instability.

UNSTEADINESS

Patients may complain of instability of gait, or an uncertainness when they walk. This is usually separable from vertigo and light-headedness. It is commonly due to a multifactorial disorder in one or more systems: visual, vestibular, dorsal column, or auditory. Elderly patients commonly have this complaint, and often have poor vision, limited hearing, and decreased vibration, which is possibly complicated by the de-afferentation that comes with bilateral knee replacement. Treatment for this disorder is fixing whatever sensory deficit can be fixed, and therapies that condition the vestibular and balance systems to movements of various kinds.

WOOZINESS

Vertigo can be caused by psychogenic factors or by hyperventilation. In a study of a large series of patients who complained of dizziness, one of the most common causes was hyperventilation. Patients
with somatoform disorders and phobias also may complain of dizziness. Often patients of this type agree that their feeling represents
"wooziness." An extensive examination for nystagmus and positional vertigo is appropriate. In addition, hyperventilation of the
patient for 2 to 4 minutes may reproduce his or her symptoms and
be therapeutically helpful.

Occasionally, despite careful evaluation, a patient's dizziness
appears to be idiopathic. In these circumstances, symptomatic
treatment and careful follow-up of the patient are required.

APPENDIX: TYPES OF BENIGN POSITIONAL NYSTAGMUS

1. Posterior semicircular canal canalithiasis: 90% of all BPPV.
   Delayed by a few seconds (latent), peaks in 20 to 30 seconds
   and then decays, complete resolution with maintained posture
   (habituation). Torsional with a vertical component. May get
   reversed nystagmus when brought to upright posture. Beats
   towards downward ear (geotropic). Reduced with repeated
   precipitation (fatigable).
2. Horizontal semicircular canal: purely horizontal, geotropic
   (beating towards downward ear), asymmetric. Direction reverses
   with change in head position from one side to other. Intensity of
   nystagmus greater with head rotated to involved side.
3. Anterior canal BPPV: rare, rotatory, vertical component beating downward. Cupulolithiasis (otoconia adherent to the
   cupula): with posterior canal form, nystagmus is geotropic,
   nonlatent, intense, long lasting, and nonfatigable.

Suggested Readings

Chawla N, Olshaker JS. Diagnosis and management of dizziness
    and vertigo. *Med Clin North Am.* 2006;90:291–304.
Cutrer FM, Baloh RW. Migraine-associated dizziness. *Headache.*
    1992;32:300–304.
Dieterich M. Dizziness. *Neurologist.* 2004;10:154–164.
Korres S, Balatsouras DG, Ferekidis E. Prognosis of patients with
    benign paroxysmal positional vertigo treated with repositioning
    maneuvers. *J Laryngol Otol.* 2006;120:528–533.
Thirlwall AS, Kundu S. Diuretics for Ménière's disease or syn-
    drome. *Cochrane Database Syst Rev.* 2006;3:CD003599.

Hyperreflexia

Normal reflexes suggest that the motor system is functioning appropriately. The main motor pathway, the corticospinal tract, descends from the cortex to different segments of the spinal cord. Neurons in this tract are upper motor neurons; the tract is also known as the pyramidal tract. The upper motor neurons synapse with lower motor neurons in the anterior gray matter of the spinal cord at the root level where the lower motor neuron exits. The corticospinal tract travels from the motor cortex through the internal capsule, and down the cerebral peduncles in the midbrain; it passes through the anterior pons, then crosses in the pyramids of the medulla, and follows the lateral corticospinal tract in the spinal cord.

The lateral corticospinal tract crosses in the pyramids of the medulla.

Pathologically hyperactive reflexes imply disease in the corticospinal tract; an upper motor neuron disorder. Other signs of upper motor neuron disorder include spasticity, clonus, slow motor movements, and weakness of certain muscle groups (deltoid, triceps, wrist and finger extensors, hip flexors, knee flexors, and ankle dorsiflexors and evertors). An upgoing toe (a positive Babinski response) is a cardinal manifestation of upper motor neuron dysfunction. In the acute phase of an upper motor neuron lesion, hyporeflexia often is present, with hyperreflexia slowly developing over 1 to 2 weeks.

Babinski response: When the lateral border of the sole is stroked with a sharp edge (e.g., a broken tongue depressor) from the heel to the base of the small toe, the great toe goes up (dorsiflexes, extends). Normally, in adults the toe goes down. In infants, the toes go up until this reflex is suppressed (Fig. 7.1).

UNILATERAL HYPERREFLEXIA

Unilateral hyperreflexia or a unilateral upgoing toe implies upper motor neuron injury on one side of the nervous system (same side of the spinal cord or the opposite side of brainstem, internal capsule, or cortex). Decide whether this represents an old lesion that

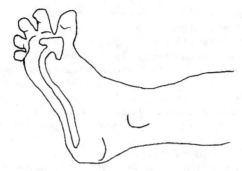

FIGURE 7.1. Babinski sign. The toe goes up with a sharp stimulus to the lateral border of the sole of the foot.

does not require further investigation or a newly developing one. You will need to check for the following:

1. *History of birth injury.* An otherwise normal person may have unilateral hyperreflexia with no apparent cause. The unilateral hyperreflexia may be a result of birth injury with mild cerebral palsy.
2. *Old neurologic disease.* A patient with a history of meningitis, stroke, subdural hematoma, or other injury may have unilateral hyperreflexia. A small stroke may not have been recognized by the patient.
3. *Asymptomatic cervical cord disease.* This disease commonly causes unilateral or bilateral hyperreflexia in older people.
4. *Newly developing signs or symptoms.* If the history suggests this, a full investigation is warranted.

Note: Unilateral corticospinal tract signs may be subtle. Look for a mild pronator drift, slowing of fine motor movements on one side, a tendency to flex the arm while walking, and the inability to roll the arms alternately around each other. In a unilateral disorder, the good arm may roll around the paretic arm.

Pronator drift: With the arms outstretched and palm turned up, the affected arm tends to drift down and the thumb turns inward.

BILATERAL HYPERREFLEXIA

Bilateral hyperreflexia with upgoing toes implies bilateral pyramidal tract dysfunction. Note the following:

1. Consider *spinal cord compression* as a cause. Ask about a sensory loss, bowel and bladder dysfunction, back pain, or weakness in the legs. Check for a sensory level, motor level, local back tenderness or deformity, or a lax sphincter (see Chapter 9).

2. *Cervical spondylosis* is the most common cause of spinal cord dysfunction in the elderly. Ask about neck pain, weakness, or paresthesias in the arms. Check for hyperreflexia, muscle wasting in the arms, radicular sensory changes in the arms, decreased range of motion of the neck, and degenerative changes on radiograph of the cervical spine.

3. *Multiple sclerosis* (MS) is an important cause of hyperreflexia in young and middle-aged patients. Establish whether there are "multiple lesions in time and space." If MS is suspected, obtain brain magnetic resonance imaging (see Chapter 21).

4. *Multiple small strokes* (état lacunaire) can cause bilateral hyperreflexia, and are frequently seen in the elderly with hypertension or diabetes. Check for a history of multiple small strokes (although they may have been clinically silent) and for other evidence of vascular disease (e.g., bruits, decreased peripheral pulses). Search for other signs of "multiple stroke" syndrome: emotional lability, brisk jaw jerk, increased gag reflex, and ataxia (features of pseudobulbar palsy).

5. *Familial spastic paraparesis* may present with slowly progressive, bilateral hyperreflexia and spasticity. Check for a family history and high arched feet. Leukodystrophies may have similar signs. Human T-lymphotropic virus type 1 (HTLV-I) infection also may cause spastic paraparesis.

6. *Metabolic causes of hyperreflexia* include hepatic and uremic encephalopathy, vitamin B_{12} deficiency, and adrenoleukodystrophies. Recently copper deficiency myelopathy has been seen in patients after gastric bypass surgery (known as "swayback").

7. *Amyotrophic lateral sclerosis* (ALS) causes increased reflexes caused by pyramidal tract involvement in the brainstem or spinal cord. Brainstem (corticobulbar) involvement causes brisk jaw jerk, hyperactive gag reflex, dysarthria, and dysphagia. Patients may have a Babinski reflex, spasticity, and weakness consistent with an upper motor neuron pattern. In addition, anterior horn cell (lower motor neuron) involvement causes fasciculations, wasting, and weakness often most prominent in the arms. The combination of upper and lower motor neuron signs in spinal cord and brainstem without sensory loss is virtually diagnostic of ALS, particularly with bulbar or pseudobulbar involvement.

8. *Hyperreflexia can be seen in otherwise normal, anxious patients.*

HYPERREFLEXIA IN THE LEGS ONLY

Hyperreflexia in both arms and legs implies a lesion at the cervical cord or higher; *hyperreflexia in the legs* implies a lesion below the cervical cord. Lesions in the thoracic cord include tumors, disc protrusions, trauma, and vascular malformations.

Note that sometimes hyperreflexia occurs in the legs from lesions above the thoracic region.

1. In *cerebral palsy*, leg fibers may be selectively involved in the white matter of the hemispheres, giving increased reflexes in the legs only ("spastic diparesis").
2. *Cervical spinal stenosis* may present with only leg weakness and spasticity, with relatively few symptoms of arm or neck involvement.
3. By virtue of their location, *parasagittal intracranial masses* may affect cortical leg fibers producing hyperreflexia in legs only, mimicking a cord lesion. Headache, seizures, papilledema, or personality change may be present.
4. *Hydrocephalus* may present with spastic paraparesis, because parasagittal leg fibers are stretched most by dilated lateral ventricles.
5. *Arnold-Chiari malformation* with cerebellar tonsillar ectopia, and brainstem deformity may be associated with a spastic paraparesis.

Suggested Readings

Chouinard PA, Paus T. The primary and premotor areas of the human cerebral cortex. *Neuroscientist.* 2006;12:143–152.

Emery SE. Diagnosis and treatment of cervical spondylotic myelopathy. *J Am Acad Orthop Surg.* 2001;6:376–388.

Van Gijn J. The Babinski sign: the first hundred years. *J Neurol.* 1996;243:675–683.

8 Hyporeflexia/Peripheral Neuropathy

Hypoactive reflexes are caused by disease between the spinal cord and muscle, typically involving the root, plexus, or peripheral nerves. Reduced reflexes indicate that one or more components of the reflex pathway are abnormal: peripheral nerve, sensory root, anterior horn cells in cord, motor roots, or muscle. Disturbances of any part of the reflex arc may cause hyporeflexia. Reflexes can be reinforced by having patients pull their hands apart or bite down while the reflex is tested (the Jendrassik maneuver). Patients voluntarily tensing their muscles will diminish or extinguish the reflex, and may need to be distracted. Areflexia implies no reflexes, even with reinforcement. Reflexes present only with reinforcement imply an intact reflex pathway and may or may not be abnormal. Consider the following points when confronted with hyporeflexia:

1. *Normally hypoactive reflexes.* Occasionally, normal individuals may have hyporeflexia with no other obvious cause. The presence of a reflex with reinforcement and absence of other signs are reassuring.
2. *Delayed relaxation phase of the reflex.* This unique hypoactive or "hung up" reflex is classic for hypothyroidism and at times serves as the first clue to this metabolic abnormality. It is best seen in the ankle jerk reflex.
3. *Asymptomatic areflexia with a large pupil.* This is a benign syndrome (Adie syndrome), consisting of generalized areflexia with a large pupil that reacts to accommodation but only slowly to direct light.
4. *Myopathy.* Muscle disorders may cause hyporeflexia but usually not areflexia. The decrease in reflex is consistent with the degree of muscle wasting and weakness. Remember, weakness from muscle disease is generally more marked proximally (shoulder and hip), whereas weakness from peripheral nerve disease is more marked distally (hand and foot). Neuromuscular junction disorders usually spare the reflexes.
5. *Isolated unilaterally absent reflex.* This important sign of disc disease compressing spinal roots can be seen with diseases affecting specific peripheral nerves (see Chapter 10).

Remember, *mononeuropathy and plexus injuries*, whether traumatic or from tumor, are other important causes of asymmetric reflex loss (see Chapter 10).

6. *Bilateral areflexia* is a key sign of neuropathy (discussed later).
   A patient with no reflexes usually has a neuropathy. Similarly,
   a neuropathy that is "length-dependent," in that the part of the
   nerve furthest from the cell body is most affected, may cause
   absent ankle jerks as an early sign.

PERIPHERAL NEUROPATHY

Peripheral neuropathies occur in a broad category of diseases,
many of which are common and treatable. The key manifestations
include bilateral or multifocal hyporeflexia, sensory or motor
involvement, and (at times) autonomic dysfunction.

Peripheral neuropathies are characterized in a variety of ways,
which may help in establishing their etiology. The temporal profile may be acute, subacute, or chronic. The pattern may be distal
or proximal, symmetric or asymmetric, diffuse or multifocal. The
nerve fibers involved may be sensory, motor, autonomic, or a combination thereof. The pathology may be axonal (involving
the nerve itself), demyelinating (involving the nerve sheath), or a
combination. It may be vasculitic (inflammation to the blood vessels supplying the nerve causing nerve injury) or neuronal (involving the cell body). The fiber type may be large fiber (vibration and
position sense) or small fiber (pin, temperature, and autonomic
involvement).

The history and physical examination often help to establish
possible etiologies. For example, a rapidly progressive course with
areflexia, vibration loss, and proximal and distal weakness occurring after a viral illness suggests an acute demyelinating inflammatory polyneuropathy. A slow course with distal muscle wasting in
the feet, distal pin and vibration loss, and loss of ankle jerks suggests a chronic, axonal sensorimotor polyneuropathy.

ACUTE AREFLEXIA WITH WEAKNESS

Acute areflexia, with weakness and little sensory loss. This is the classic presentation of acute inflammatory demyelinating polyneuropathy (AIDP), or *Guillain–Barré syndrome*. This may follow a
systemic infection or vaccination by days or weeks, or it may occur
after an event such as a surgery.

Clinical Characteristics

It is typical to have progressive weakness over a few days, with gait unsteadiness, arm weakness, and facial and respiratory involvement, sometimes with an "ascending" pattern. With severe weakness, ventilatory assistance may be necessary. A form in which cranial nerve involvement predominates is called the Miller–Fisher variant (characterized by ophthalmoparesis, ataxia, and areflexia). Autonomic dysfunction may occur, causing bladder dysfunction and fluctuations of blood pressure, heart rate, and temperature. Usually, the disease is monophasic and patients recover, although the recovery may take months in severely affected patients.

Diagnosis

Clinical features include rapidly progressive muscle weakness of proximal and distal muscles, areflexia, mild distal sensory loss, and bifacial weakness. Cerebrospinal fluid (CSF) initially may be normal, but over days it shows an increase in protein with few or no white cells. Nerve conduction studies also may be normal initially, but they ultimately show evidence of a demyelinating polyneuropathy.

Treatment

Because of the potential for respiratory failure and dangerous autonomic fluctuations, careful monitoring of respiratory and cardiac function is mandatory once the diagnosis is made. Vital capacity and negative inspiratory force are useful in studying respiratory function and predicting the need for ventilator assistance. Treatment to avoid decubiti, pressure palsies, deep vein thrombosis, and other intensive care unit (ICU) complications is important. Plasmapheresis has been shown in large randomized studies to shorten the duration of illness, especially ICU course and time in hospital. Intravenous gamma globulin (IVIG) may be of equal benefit. Unless severe axonal injury occurs, a complete or near-complete recovery is expected in weeks or months.

Differential Diagnosis

Other causes of acute symmetric motor weakness that may mimic AIDP include acute intermittent porphyria, tick paralysis, Lyme disease, acquired immunodeficiency virus (AIDS), botulism, toxin exposure, diphtheria (palatal and extraocular muscle palsies), and polyarteritis. Think of polio in unimmunized children. West Nile virus may cause a poliomyelitis picture. A slower course or a relapsing picture suggests chronic inflammatory demyelinating polyneuropathy (CIDP), which is treated with prednisone or IVIG.

AREFLEXIA WITH SENSORY INVOLVEMENT AND LITTLE OR LATE-DEVELOPING MOTOR LOSS

A variety of systemic illnesses may cause predominantly a sensory neuropathy that may progress over weeks to years. Consider the following:

1. *Diabetes*. Various neuropathies may be associated with diabetes (see Chapter 22).
2. *Alcoholism* (neuropathy is the result of a nutritional deficit). These patients have a sensory neuropathy, often painful, involving feet and hands, including decreased vibration sense (see Chapter 27).
3. *Vitamin B$_{12}$ deficiency*. This may cause a sensory neuropathy often associated with spinal cord involvement. Characteristic findings include loss of vibration and position sense, distal reflex loss, paresthesias, and upgoing toes.
4. *Medications*. Cis-platinum and other medications may cause a predominantly sensory neuropathy. Other medications that can cause neuropathy include metronidazole, phenytoin, many agents used against HIV, and occasionally statins.
5. *Uremia*. Patients with uremia may have sensory or sensorimotor involvement with "restless" leg symptoms and burning paresthesias (see Chapter 26).
6. *Malignancy*. A malignancy (especially lung cancer) may have a sensory neuropathy as the presenting complaint as part of a paraneoplastic syndrome.
7. *Amyloidosis*. This disease, either primary or secondary to another systemic illness, may cause a sensory and autonomic neuropathy, preferentially affecting small fibers (pain, temperature, sweating loss, trophic changes).
8. *Sjögren syndrome*. This common and under-recognized rheumatologic condition may be associated with a predominantly sensory syndrome of ataxia, limb involvement, and subacute to chronic course. Ask about dry eyes, dry mouth, and arthritic symptoms. Patients may have prominent facial sensory loss, because this is often due to loss of dorsal root ganglion cells and not dependent on fiber length.

Note: A familial sensory radicular neuropathy with autosomal dominant inheritance may present during the second and third decades. Fabry and Refsum diseases may present as sensory neuropathy.

MULTIFOCAL PATTERN WITH ASYMMETRIC MOTOR AND SENSORY INVOLVEMENT

This pattern may be seen with demyelinating neuropathies and with vasculitic neuropathies. Vasculitis, diabetes, sarcoidosis, Lyme disease, leprosy, and AIDS are disorders to consider. Tomaculous neuropathy is a familial disorder with multiple compression palsies (i.e., median at the wrist, ulnar at the elbow, peroneal at the knee).

1. *Chronic, distal, relatively symmetric motor and sensory neuropathy.* This is the most common pattern of neuropathy. Often it is caused by diabetes mellitus, and is seen with many other systemic disorders, such as nutritional deficits, toxins, uremia, hypothyroidism, dysproteinemias, collagen vascular diseases, and paraneoplastic conditions.
2. *Bilateral areflexia and neuropathy on a familial basis.* The prototype for familial neuropathy is *Charcot–Marie–Tooth* disease (peroneal muscular atrophy). These patients have sensory loss, "champagne-bottle" legs, a widespread areflexia not merely confined to the ankles, and pes cavus. Familial neuropathies may be associated with other inherited neurologic diseases and accompanied by other signs (e.g., tremor, nystagmus, optic atrophy).
3. *Predominantly motor neuropathy.* Amyotrophic lateral sclerosis is the archetype; however, some paraneoplastic and toxic neuropathies also may be predominantly motor. Check for antibodies to GM1 and MAG. Porphyria may present as an acute motor neuropathy. Nerve conduction studies will help define those that spare the sensory fibers.
4. *Autonomic neuropathy.* This may be seen with diabetes or alcoholism, or as a paraneoplastic syndrome, and it may occur with toxins and amyloidosis. An acute autonomic neuropathy also has been described as a post-infectious complication. Familial autonomic neuropathies include Riley–Day syndrome. Symptoms include orthostatic hypotension, sweating abnormalities, gastrointestinal (GI) symptoms, impotence, and bladder dysfunction.

WORKUP OF NEUROPATHIES

In some cases, the clinical history and examination will define the etiology of the neuropathy without extensive investigation. In other instances, a directed workup, keeping in mind the type of neuropathy and possible etiologies, is required for a diagnosis. In some instances, no diagnosis emerges despite extensive workup (most commonly in chronic distal sensorimotor axonal neuropathies).

Check these important points when dealing with a neuropathic process of undetermined cause:

1. Is there evidence of toxin exposure (painful red feet, GI disturbances), such as thallium (alopecia), lead (affects upper extremities, including motor neuropathies with wrist drop, and causes lead line in gums), or other metals (copper, zinc, mercury)? Consider organic toxins and occupational exposures.
2. Check for drugs that may cause neuropathy. Nitrofurantoin, isoniazid, vincristine, and cisplatinum are common offenders. Look up each medication and any "herbal" medications that the patient takes.
3. Does the patient have an associated systemic illness: hypothyroidism, syphilis, amyloid (large tongue, GI symptoms), myeloma or other gammopathy, leprosy (anesthetic skin patches), lupus, AIDS, Lyme disease, sarcoidosis, polyarteritis, pernicious anemia, porphyria, diabetes, renal failure, rheumatoid arthritis, Sjögren syndrome, or systemic sclerosis?
4. Is the neuropathy relapsing? CIDP, alcohol, lead, or porphyria may be the cause.
5. Electromyography and nerve conduction studies assist in establishing the presence of neuropathy (characterizing the pattern as predominantly axonal, demyelinating, or multifocal; motor or sensory; large fiber or small fiber) and may give clues to possible etiologies.
6. Nerve biopsy is useful only in a small group of patients, and in many cases is nonspecific. It is most beneficial when considering a demyelinating neuropathy, vasculitis, amyloidosis, or sarcoidosis.
7. Spinal fluid is usually nondiagnostic, but may show increased protein in inflammatory neuropathies, diabetes, and neuropathies associated with cancer. Any neuropathy affecting the proximal root may increase CSF protein.
8. Consider testing for paraneoplastic antibodies in patients with unusual neuropathies without other apparent cause, especially

with systemic problems such as weight loss and malaise (see Chapter 23). A rare condition called POEMS causes peripheral neuropathy, organomegaly, endocrinopathy, and monoclonal gammopathy. Skin changes are occasionally seen.

TREATMENT OF NEUROPATHIES

Treatment depends on the etiology, removal of the offending toxin or drug, treatment of the underlying systemic illness, or treatment of a specific remediable neuropathy. Vitamin supplementation may be helpful, particularly in nutritional neuropathies. Immunosuppression may be useful in immunologically mediated neuropathies. Rehabilitative devices and avoidance of pressure palsies are helpful in some neuropathies. The treatment of painful neuropathies is reviewed in Chapter 29.

Suggested Readings

Chalk CH. Acquired peripheral neuropathy. *Neurol Clin.* 1997;15:501–528.

Dyck PJ, Dyck JB, Chalk CH. The 10 P's: a mnemonic helpful in characterization and differential diagnosis of peripheral neuropathy. *Neurology.* 1992;42:14–18.

Dyck PJ, Dyck JB, Grant IA, et al. Ten steps in characterizing and diagnosing patients with peripheral neuropathy. *Neurology.* 1996;47:10–17.

Hughes RA, Wijdicks EF, Barohn R, et al. Practice parameter: immunotherapy for Guillain-Barré syndrome: report of the Quality Standards Subcommittee of the American Academy of Neurology. *Neurology.* 2003;61:736–740.

Hughes RA, Wijdicks EF, Benson E, et al. Supportive care for patients with Guillain-Barré syndrome. *Arch Neurol.* 2005;62:1194–1198.

Poncelet AN. An algorithm for the evaluation of peripheral neuropathy. *Am Fam Physician.* 1998;57:755–764.

Spinal Cord Compression

CASE

A 64-year-old woman with known multiple myeloma has a 1-week history of sharp back pain radiating around the left costal margin that is worse with coughing. For the past day she has noticed incontinence of urine, and during the past 5 hours she has become weak in her legs. Dexamethasone is given intravenously, and emergency magnetic resonance imaging (MRI) of the spine shows an epidural mass at T6, with cord compression.

Diagnosis

Acute spinal cord compression, T6, caused by epidural bony metastasis.

Acute spinal cord compression is a neurologic emergency. Prognosis is related to the delay between onset of neurologic symptoms and treatment. Being alert to the possibility of cord compression is crucial for early diagnosis.

Characteristic symptoms include back pain; root pain, often radiating around the side or down a limb; paresthesias in legs ("funny feelings," tingling, or numbness); change in urine function (patient urinates more or less frequently or is incontinent); weakness in lower extremities (especially when climbing stairs); and constipation or fecal incontinence.

Note that the earlier diagnosis and treatment are started with spinal cord compression, the better the outcome. Have a high index of suspicion for anyone with back pain and sensory symptoms in the legs.

EARLY SIGNS

1. Loss of pinprick sensation or a different reaction to pinprick in the lower extremities. The patient may have a sensory "level" to pinprick. There may be a temperature "level" to a cool object, or a "sweat" level.
2. Altered position or vibration sensation below the level of the lesion.

3. Tenderness over the spine is a helpful sign in determining the level of the lesion.
4. Hyperreflexia below the level of the lesion. If the lesion is in the thoracic cord, legs are hyperreflexic compared with arms.
5. Signs are usually bilateral (i.e., both legs, both arms) rather than unilateral.

LATE SIGNS

1. Definite weakness.
2. Definite hyperreflexia.
3. Upgoing toes.
4. A sensory level to pinprick, temperature, or vibration. It is often helpful to check vibration sense up and down the spine in search of a level. Check for a sweat level.
5. Loss of anal sphincter tone and voluntary contraction, absent abdominal reflexes, and absent bulbocavernosus reflex.
6. Urinary retention, or incontinence of bowel or bladder.
7. Loss of superficial abdominal reflexes.

CAUSES OF SPINAL CORD COMPRESSION

Epidural Compression

1. Metastatic tumor (especially from lung, breast, and prostate). Spinal cord compression may be the initial manifestation of malignancy.
2. Trauma.
3. Lymphoma.
4. Multiple myeloma.
5. Epidural abscess or hematoma.
6. Cervical or thoracic disc protrusion, spondylosis or spondylolisthesis.
7. Atlantoaxial subluxation (rheumatoid arthritis).

Extramedullary, Intradural Compression

1. Meningioma.
2. Neurofibroma.

Intramedullary Expansion

1. Glioma.
2. Ependymoma.
3. Arteriovenous malformation.

DIAGNOSTIC STEPS

1. Perform a careful neurologic examination and estimate the level of the cord lesion. Note that the lesion may lie above the sensory level, because of partial injury and lamination of sensory tracts. Also note that the dermatomal level does not correspond to the bony level because of the termination of the cord at about T12-L1 (Fig. 9.1).

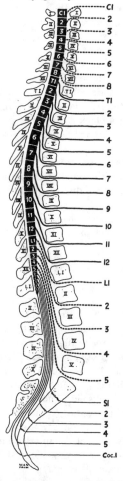

FIGURE 9.1. Spinal cord segments and their respective nerve roots. (Reproduced with permission from Haymaker W, Woodhall B. *Peripheral Nerve Injuries*. Philadelphia: Saunders; 1945.)

2. Check for primary tumor sites (e.g., careful examination of breast, nodes, and prostate; chest radiograph; and routine laboratory studies, including complete blood count, liver function test, and prostate specific antigen). Consider at a later time further imaging with CT chest, abdomen, pelvis, PET scanning, but do not delay treatment for such investigations.

3. Plain films of the spine may reveal (i) vertebral collapse or subluxation, (ii) bony erosion secondary to tumor, or (iii) calcification (meningioma).

4. Urgent consultation with a neurologist or neurosurgeon, and a radiation therapist is needed.

5. Perform an MRI scan of the spine with sagittal cuts through the entire spine and axial cuts through suspicious areas. If the patient cannot tolerate an MRI, a computed tomographic myelogram usually is done. MRI has become the diagnostic study of choice in acute cord compression. If myelography is necessary and if a spinal block is seen on myelogram, image above the block using a cisternal puncture to examine the extent of disease.

6. Do not perform a lumbar puncture if cord compression is suspected; **patients with spinal cord compression may worsen after lumbar puncture due to shifting mass after pressure changes.**

7. Image the entire spine if possible. There may be multiple sites of compression, which influences therapy.

TREATMENT

Treatment depends on the site(s) of cord injury and the etiology. Treatment is most effective if instituted early. Acute bowel and bladder dysfunction in the setting of cord compression is an emergency, as is rapidly progressive weakness. Modalities include radiotherapy (for such disorders as metastatic breast or prostate cancer, or Hodgkin lymphoma); surgical decompression for solitary radioresistant, extradural solid tumors; or a combination of both. A single randomized trial indicated that a combination of surgical decompression and radiotherapy was superior to radiotherapy alone (level 1b). A dose of dexamethasone (16–60 mg intravenously) is usually given immediately when compression is suspected, because clinically it may help to preserve spinal cord function. A dose of dexamethasone should be continued into radiotherapy and then tapered.

DIFFERENTIAL DIAGNOSIS OF NONCOMPRESSIVE SPINAL CORD INJURY

1. *Transverse myelitis* is characterized by the acute or subacute development of paraplegia or quadriplegia, occasionally asymmetric, associated with back pain and sensory loss. It may be related to a preceding viral illness (e.g., mononucleosis). The cerebrospinal fluid may show pleocytosis with increased protein and normal sugar levels. Studies for disorders such as Lyme disease, lupus erythematosus, syphilis, human immunodeficiency virus, cytomegalovirus, and herpes simplex virus should be considered. MRI is usually necessary to rule out a compressive lesion. In addition, MRI may show intramedullary pathology such as a plaque of demyelinating disease. Treatment is supportive. Corticosteroids often are used when the etiology is thought to be post-infectious or demyelinating. Consider assessment for Devic disease (neuromyelitis optica).

2. *Radiation myelopathy* usually occurs 6 months to 5 years after irradiation to the thoracic area of the spinal cord (e.g., for lymphoma). Onset may be insidious or abrupt, and may be limited to paresthesias, or progress to paralysis. MRI or myelography is needed to rule out a compressive lesion and may show intrinsic cord abnormalities. There is no known treatment, and the myelopathy is probably secondary to vascular damage to the spinal cord. Steroids or anticoagulants have been tried in such cases with varied results.

3. *Acute myelopathy* also may be secondary to toxins (e.g., heroin, arsenic), associated with malignancy elsewhere in the body. This can be a remote effect, or secondary to vascular infarction of the spinal cord caused by anterior spinal artery occlusion. In the latter condition, motor function, pain, and temperature appreciation are affected, whereas position and vibration sense (posterior column functions) are spared.

4. Acute spinal cord trauma is treated with stabilization of the spine, and with methylprednisolone according to a specific infusion protocol depending on the time after injury.

SPINAL CORD TRACTS

It is useful to understand the major tracts that descend and ascend through the spinal cord. See Figure 34.10 for the cross-sectional anatomy of the cervical spinal cord.

Descending Tracts

The descending motor fibers travel in the spinal cord primarily in the lateral corticospinal tract. Some descend in the anterior corticospinal tract as well. The lateral corticospinal track crosses in the lower medulla and descends in the lateral cord to synapse with the lower motor neuron. Thus a lesion on the left cord would cause weakness on the left side.

Ascending Tracts

The spinothalamic tract carries pain, temperature, and tickle sensation from the contralateral limbs and body. Sensory fibers enter the spinal cord and synapse with second-order neurons in the dorsal root. These fibers then cross over two or three segments to the opposite side of the cord in the anterior commissure, which is in the anterior deep cord just in front of the central canal. They travel in the spinothalamic tract to the thalamus, where they relay with third-order neurons. Thus a lesion in the left spinal cord would cause pain and temperature loss on the right side of the body two or three cord segments below the level of the lesion.

The dorsal columns carry primarily two-point discrimination and light touch (possibly vibration) up to the sensory cortex. These also enter in the dorsal root, but travel on the same side of the spinal cord in the dorsal columns. They synapse with second-order neurons in the medulla. These neurons cross the midline in the medulla in the internal arcuate fibers to synapse in the opposite thalamus. The third-order neurons travel to the sensory cortex. Thus, a lesion in the left spinal cord causes a loss of two-point discrimination in the ipsilateral body below the lesion.

■ Brown–Séquard Syndrome

A hemicord transsection such as might be seen with a gunshot wound to the spinal cord would thus cause ipsilateral weakness below the lesion (corticospinal tract), contralateral pain, and temperature loss 2 to 3 cord segments below the lesion (spinothalamic tract), and ipsilateral loss of two-point discrimination (dorsal columns). Bowel and bladder function is usually spared in such a syndrome, as bilateral injury is usually needed to cause difficulty with these functions.

Suggested Readings

Loblaw DA, Perry J, Chambers A, et al. Systematic review of the diagnosis and management of malignant extradural spinal cord compression: the Cancer Care Ontario practice guidelines initiative's neuro-oncology disease site group. *J Clin Oncol.* 2005;23:2028–2037.

Patchell RA, Tibbs PA, Regine WF, et al. Direct decompressive surgical resection in the treatment of spinal cord compression caused by metastatic cancer: a randomised trial. *Lancet.* 2005;366:643–648.

Scott TF, Kassab SL, Pittock SJ. Neuromyelitis optica IgG status in acute partial transverse myelitis. *Arch Neurol.* 2006;63:1398–1400.

Transverse myelitis consortium working group. Proposed diagnostic criteria and nosology of acute transverse myelitis. *Neurology.* 2002;59: 499–505.

Wagner R, Jagoda A. Spinal cord syndromes. *Emerg Med Clin North Am.* 1997;15:699–711.

10 Peripheral Nerve and Root Dysfunction

CASE

A 16-year-old male, right-handed high school student is out for the very first time with a girl at a double feature. He has his arm around her and even though it hurts, he doesn't want to move it. After the show is over, he finds he has aching pain in the mid-humerus and cannot extend his wrist or fingers.

Diagnosis

Saturday night palsy; radial nerve palsy in the spiral groove.

To diagnose peripheral nerve and root injuries, one must determine which muscles are affected, outline the territory of sensory loss, and note any reflex changes. One then compares this distribution with the known territories supplied by nerves or roots to localize the lesion.

REFLEXES

Reflexes are diminished in root and peripheral nerve disease. There are four primary reflexes to remember, along with the particular roots and muscles necessary for their function. An easy way to learn the roots is to remember that going from ankle to triceps, the roots are numbered consecutively from 1 to 8 (Table 10.1).

ROOTS AND MUSCLES

Each muscle is supplied by two or more roots. Thus, weakness associated with injury to only one root is partial; as opposed to peripheral nerve injury, which may cause complete muscle weakness. Nevertheless, certain muscles tend to be preferentially supplied by certain roots, so that they are particularly affected by injury to the root. Table 10.2 describes the most useful muscles to

■ **TABLE 10.1. Four Primary Reflexes**

Reflex	Roots	Muscle
Ankle jerk	S1	Gastrocnemius
Knee jerk	(L2, L3) L4	Quadriceps
Biceps	C5, C6	Biceps
Triceps	C7 (C8)	Triceps

test for root injury, and which roots supply each muscle. Each root has a sensory distribution as represented on the standard dermatome chart (see Chapter 34). The most useful root dermatomes to remember are:

- C2—over the posterior head.
- C4—the shoulder.
- C7—the middle finger.
- T4—the nipple.
- T10—the umbilicus.
- L3—the knee.
- S1—the lateral foot.
- S3, S4, and S5—the anal region.

■ **TABLE 10.2. Roots and the Primary Muscles They Supply**

Root	Muscle	Action
C5	Deltoid	Shoulder abduction
C5	Infraspinatus	Humeral external rotation
C5, C6	Biceps	Flexion of the supinated forearm
C6	Extensor carpi radialis and ulnaris	Wrist extension
C7	Extensors digitorum	Finger extensions; forearm extension at elbow
C7	Triceps	Elbow extension
C8, T1	Interossei and lumbricals	Digital abduction and adduction
L2-4	Quadriceps, iliopsoas	Knee extension, thigh on hip flexion
	Adductor group	Thigh adduction
L5	Anterior tibial and extensor hallucis	Ankle and large toe dorsiflexion
S1	Gastrocnemius	Ankle plantar flexion

NERVES AND MUSCLES OF THE UPPER EXTREMITIES

Median Nerve

The median nerve (C6-T1) originates in the brachial plexus, and supplies two basic muscle groups:

1. *Forearm:* pronator of the forearm, radial flexion, and wrist abduction.
2. *Hand:* the first two Lumbricales (index and middle finger flexion at the metacarpophalangeal joint), thumb Opposition with opponens pollicis, Abduction with abductor pollicis brevis, and Flexion with flexor pollicis brevis ("LOAF" muscles). *Sensory loss* involves the thumb, index, and middle fingers and half of the ring finger (Fig. 10.1).

Clinical comment: A complete median nerve lesion (forearm and hand muscles) is usually secondary to traumatic injury in the axilla, or to a lesion affecting the median nerve at the elbow. Entrapment of the anterior interosseus branch causes weakness of thumb distal flexion, and flexion of the distal phalanx of the second and third digits. Entrapment at the wrist is common after wrist fractures. A clinical syndrome of median entrapment at the wrist with intermittent or progressive symptoms is called "carpal tunnel syndrome." Patients with this syndrome often complain of numbness and tingling in the thumb and first two fingers. The hands typically "fall asleep" with use or at night (nocturnal paresthesias). The earliest weakness is a difficulty twisting jar lids open or a tendency to drop objects. Muscle wasting and obvious loss of

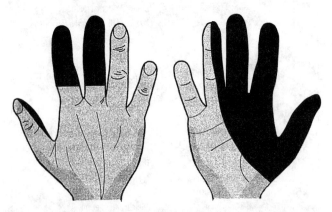

FIGURE 10.1. Median sensory loss.

power occurs later. The diagnosis may be confirmed by nerve conduction studies. Carpal tunnel syndrome is often bilateral and may be associated with systemic processes; consider rheumatoid arthritis, hypothyroidism, diabetes, pregnancy, gout, acromegaly, and amyloidosis. Medical management includes treating the underlying disease, splinting the wrist, and injecting steroids into the carpal tunnel region. A single injection of steroids is beneficial in terms of pain and function at 3 months, but additional injections do not seem to be beneficial. Surgical decompression of the carpal tunnel may be necessary and is usually successful.

Ulnar Nerve

The ulnar nerve (C8-T1) supplies muscles and sensory areas on the palm not supplied by the median nerve. When ulnar nerve disease is suspected, think of little finger and hypothenar eminence. The ulnar nerve runs in the ulnar groove at the medial aspect of the elbow ("funny bone") and supplies the following two muscle groups:

1. *Forearm:* ulnar flexion at the wrist.
2. *Hand:* little finger abduction and opposition, thumb adduction, all the interosseous muscles (used to spread fingers apart and bring together), and third and fourth lumbricales (ring and little finger flexion at the metacarpophalangeal joint). *Sensory loss* involves half of the fourth finger and the little finger (Fig. 10.2).

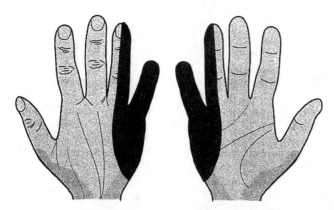

FIGURE 10.2. Ulnar sensory loss.

Clinical comment: The ulnar nerve is commonly injured at the elbow, where it is most exposed. Look for muscle weakness as opposed to the prominent sensory symptoms seen in median nerve dysfunction.

Radial Nerve

The radial nerve (C5-C8) winds around the humerus in the spiral groove, then travels in the lateral aspect of the elbow. When there is a wrist drop, think of radial nerve injury.

The radial nerve supplies these muscles:

1. *Supinator* of the forearm; the brachioradialis reflex may be lost.
2. *Extensors* of the fingers, wrist, elbow (triceps), and thumb. *Sensory loss* involves the back of the hand and is not always present (Fig. 10.3).

Clinical comment: Injury to the radial nerve may occur in the axilla (e.g., after using crutches), giving inability to extend the elbow, and may include wrist drop. If the radial nerve is involved at the humerus, only wrist drop is found. Pressure palsies are common (e.g., "bridegroom's palsy," when the groom sleeps with the bride's head on his arm).

In addition, the radial nerve is affected in diabetes and lead poisoning. In radial nerve palsy, the ability to spread the fingers apart (ulnar nerve function) may be weak because of the mechanical disadvantage caused by the wrist drop. Check with wrist resting on a flat surface (e.g., table) to overcome that handicap.

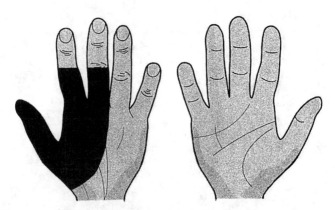

FIGURE 10.3. Radial sensory loss.

THORACIC OUTLET SYNDROME

The thoracic outlet syndrome refers to symptoms and signs that occur, because of compression of the subclavian vessels and brachial plexus at the superior aperture of the thorax between the first rib and the clavicle. Previously thought to be common, it is now clear that true neurogenic or vascular thoracic outlet syndrome is rare. Symptoms include:

1. Pain and paresthesias in the neck, shoulder, arm, and hand (C8, T1 distribution).
2. Weakness of the hand; change of color of the hand, including pallor of the fingers.
3. Aggravation of all symptoms by use of the upper limb.

Signs depend on whether primarily vascular or neural compression exists, and include supraclavicular bruit, loss or diminution of radial pulse, weakness and sensory loss in the hand, and reproduction of pain by pressure in the supraclavicular fossa or by traction on the arm. The diagnosis of thoracic outlet syndrome should be made only when definite nerve conduction or electromyogram data support the neurogenic form, or when there is evidence of vascular disease supporting the vascular form.

CERVICAL RADICULOPATHY

"Radiculopathy" refers to a disorder of an individual nerve root. A herniated disc causing nerve root compression should be suspected when there is neck pain, pain shooting down the arm ("radicular pain"), and evidence of sensory, motor, and reflex change conforming to the distribution of one or more cervical roots. Root lesions give prominent pain and sensory loss with milder weakness. This is because each muscle is supplied by two or more nerve roots, so with individual root lesions, weakness is incomplete (see Table 10.2).

CERVICAL SPONDYLOSIS

"Spondylosis" refers to degenerative aging changes of the spine. Osteophyte formation, disc degeneration, and hypertrophic changes in ligaments all are part of this process. Check for multiple, often asymmetric root involvement in the upper extremities, with muscle wasting and hypoactive reflexes in the distribution of those roots affected, and compression of the cervical spinal cord, giving hyperactive lower-extremity reflexes, upgoing toes, and leg weakness. Remember, sensory symptoms in the hands plus spastic lower extremities in patients older than age 50 years equal cervical spondylosis with myelopathy until proved otherwise. Similar symptoms may be caused by foramen magnum tumors or anomalies of the posterior fossa, such as Chiari malformations, especially in younger patients.

NERVES AND MUSCLES OF THE LOWER EXTREMITIES

Obturator Nerve

The obturator nerve (L2-L3-L4 roots, ventral portion) supplies the adductors of the thigh (brings legs together). It may be damaged during labor, involved in diabetes, or affected by local pelvic disease or by obturator hernia (Table 10.3).

Femoral Nerve

The femoral nerve (L2-L3-L4 roots, dorsal portion) supplies the iliopsoas (hip flexion), and quadriceps (knee extension). The knee jerk is diminished or absent. Numbness extends over the thigh and down the medial shin. Femoral nerve involvement may be distinguished from root involvement at L2-L3-L4 (e.g., by paravertebral tumor) by checking thigh adduction (obturator), which is affected if roots are involved, but spared if only the femoral nerve is involved. Causes of femoral neuropathy include diabetes (look for quadriceps wasting with pain over the anterior thigh), tumor, polyarteritis, pelvic trauma, and hemorrhage into the iliacus muscle in patients taking anticoagulants (retroperitoneal hematoma).

■ **TABLE 10.3. Characteristic Features Associated with Various Nerves**

Nerve	Involvement
Median	Thumb and thenar eminence
Ulnar	Little finger and hypothenar eminence
Radial	Wrist drop
Femoral	Absent knee jerk, weak hip flexion, and knee extension
Peroneal	Foot drop
Sciatic	Pain down lateral thigh and leg, often with absent ankle jerk

Lateral Femoral Cutaneous Nerve

The lateral femoral cutaneous nerve is a pure sensory nerve (L2-L3) that supplies the lateral thigh. Injury to this nerve causes tingling, burning, and pain, which is often worse with standing. The lateral femoral cutaneous nerve syndrome, "meralgia paraesthetica," is common in diabetes, and may appear during pregnancy or as a result of pressure from a tight-fitting belt, obesity, or even poor posture. Treatment involves removing the offending agent, and if necessary, injecting the nerve with steroids at its entrance to the thigh, or surgical release. A loose belt, weight loss, and non-steroidal medications are often effective treatment strategies.

Meralgia paresthetica is a common cause of unnecessary referral to neurologists.

Sciatic Nerve

The sciatic nerve (L4-S3) supplies hamstrings (flexion of the knee) and all muscles below the knee. At the knee, it divides into the *peroneal nerve*, which runs anteriorly, supplying muscles that dorsiflex and evert the foot and providing sensation on top of the foot; and the *tibial nerve*, which runs posteriorly at the knee, supplying muscles of plantar flexion, inversion, and sensation on the sole of the foot.

Clinically, the most common affliction of the sciatic nerve is "sciatica," a syndrome of pain radiating down the leg from the buttock or back. Irritation of any root from L4-S3 may produce sciatica to a varying degree. One of the most common causes of sciatica is lumbar disc protrusion (pain may be precipitated by coughing or sneezing), often with associated reflex loss and weakness in a root distribution. Straight leg raising generally aggravates the pain. Some patients may have no neurologic findings with a herniated disc, although often there is paravertebral muscle spasm. If root dysfunction occurs, this may help localize the disc protrusion level (Table 10.4). However, far lateral or far medial disc protrusions may affect the roots above or below the "usual" level, respectively (Fig. 10.4).

▓ TABLE 10.4. Most Common Lumbar Disc Syndromes				
Root	Interspace	Reflex	Weakness	Sensory
L4	L3-L4	Knee	Knee extension	Anterior thigh
L5	L4-L5	Hamstring	Invert, evert foot	Dorsum foot
S1	L5-S1	Ankle	Foot, plantar flex	Foot, lateral border

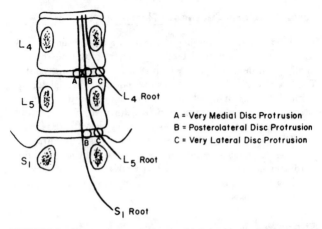

FIGURE 10.4. Disc protrusions. **A.** Very medial disc protrusion. **B.** Posterolateral disc protrusion. **C.** Very lateral disc protrusion. (From Brazis P, Masdeu JC, Biller J. *Localization in Clinical Neurology*. 5th ed. Philadelphia: Lippincott Williams & Wilkins; 2007.)

■ Treatment

Because low back pain and sciatica are frequently benign and transient, a conservative course of treatment within the first few weeks is recommended, unless there is evidence to suggest more severe dysfunction, or an unusual cause of sciatica. Instituting bed rest does not appear to be more helpful than allowing full activities. The use of pain medications or nonsteroidal medications may help in pain relief. A course of physiotherapy may be helpful. Chiropractic treatment has been shown to be as effective as medical management for acute low back pain. Epidural steroids have been shown to have only a transient effect in relieving pain from disc protrusion, and do not provide a long-term functional benefit or reduce the ultimate need for surgical treatment. If conservative management is unsuccessful, or if there is significant neurologic dysfunction, magnetic resonance imaging (MRI) or computed tomography (CT) scanning of the lumbar spine is usually effective in defining the pathology. If necessary, myelography with follow-up CT may show far lateral disc protrusions not visible on MRI. Surgical decompression of discs usually is considered when medical management fails. (For more on back pain see Chapter 29).

Peroneal Nerve

The peroneal nerve supplies dorsiflexors (tibialis anterior) and everters (turning out) of the foot. Inverters (turning in) of the foot are supplied by the tibial nerve. The sensory distribution involves the lateral aspect of the leg and dorsum of the foot.

Clinically, peroneal nerve palsy gives foot drop and is analogous to wrist drop (radial nerve) in the upper extremity. Foot drop is seen in diabetes and may be caused by trauma or pressure in a thin or wasted individual (because of the superficial location of the nerve at the head of the fibula by the knee). Hereditary peroneal neuropathy (Charcot–Marie–Tooth disease) is associated with bilateral foot drop, a wasted anterior leg compartment below the knee, and pes cavus. Remember, peroneal palsy spares the inverters of the foot. If the inverters are also weak and the lesion is higher, generally at the sciatic nerve, root, or cord level. Although peroneal palsy is the most common cause of foot drop, the differential diagnosis of foot drop includes the following:

1. Sciatic nerve injury. *Clue:* Tibialis posterior is affected, as are other muscles supplied by sciatic nerve, such as gastrocnemius.
2. L5 nerve root. *Clue:* Tibialis posterior is affected, often with associated back pain.
3. Spinal cord. *Clue:* Upper motor neuron signs (e.g., Babinski) are present.
4. Hemisphere. *Clue:* Anterior cerebral infarct causes other signs of hemiparesis and frontal lobe signs.

Posterior Tibial Nerve

The posterior tibial nerve is rarely injured alone because it runs deep in the calf. It may be entrapped distally in the tarsal tunnel, causing pain in the sole of the foot.

Conus Medullaris and Cauda Equina Lesions

The conus medullaris (lower sacral segments of the spinal cord), and cauda equina (elongated roots of the lumbar and sacral spinal nerves) can be affected by a variety of processes. Differential diagnosis includes tumor, hemorrhage, disc herniation, pelvic fracture, spondylolisthesis, and inflammatory lesions. Helpful distinguishing features are contained in Table 10.5. In either case, imaging of the lower cord and cauda equina, and possibly neurosurgical evaluation are warranted.

TABLE 10.5. Distinguishing Features of Conus Medullaris and Cauda Equina Lesions		
	Conus Medullaris	Cauda Equina
Motor weakness	Absent or mild	Usually unilateral
Sensory deficits	Bilateral (saddle)	Usually unilateral
Sphincters	Early	Late, mild

INVESTIGATION OF NERVE AND ROOT DYSFUNCTION

Examine the patient to determine whether nerves or roots are involved. Determine whether the sensory loss (or symptom) and muscle weakness (if present) fit the distribution of a particular nerve or root.

CRANIAL NERVE DISORDERS

The most useful cranial nerves to test in a clinical setting include the following:

- II—optic nerve, visual fields.
- III, IV, VI—pupil, eye movements.
- V—facial sensation, jaw movement.
- VII—facial movement, tearing, salivation.
- VIII—hearing, balance.
- IX, X—gag and swallowing.
- XII—tongue movement.

A brief review of the cranial nerves can be found in Chapter 34 (see also Fig. 34.6). More extensive reviews of cranial nerve anatomy and function can be found in textbooks of neuroanatomy.

TRIGEMINAL NEURALGIA

Excruciating, paroxysmal pain lasting seconds to minutes in the distribution of the second or third division of the fifth cranial nerve is the hallmark of trigeminal neuralgia (tic douloureux). The pain often is "triggered" by touching the side of the face, or is brought on by facial movement such as chewing. There is no objective motor or sensory loss. The cause is unknown, but may be related to a viral infection or to pressure on the nerve by a small vessel in the root entry zone. Trigeminal neuralgia is uncommon in people younger than age 40 years. When it occurs in the young patient, particularly if associated with objective sensory loss, it is frequently secondary to multiple sclerosis. Neurologic signs (loss of sensation on the face, cranial nerve palsies, long-tract signs) suggest focal pathology, such as tumor, vascular malformation, or demyelinating disease. Approximately 10% of patients with trigeminal neuralgia have a structural lesion. Treatment with carbamazepine relieves pain in most patients. Other drugs, such as oxcarbazepine and lamotrigine, may be useful. Trigeminal neuralgia refractory to medical treatment may require surgical intervention. Glycerol injection, or balloon ablation of the nerve, may be effective. Percutaneous radiofrequency coagulation of the gasserian ganglion may be effective in relieving the pain of trigeminal neuralgia. Radiosurgery may be beneficial for this syndrome. Some patients may require vascular decompression of the trigeminal nerve via craniotomy (suboccipital decompression). The latter procedure carries a 1% mortality, which appropriately limits its use.

SEVENTH-NERVE PALSIES

Peripheral involvement of the seventh cranial nerve is a well-recognized syndrome. Onset may be heralded by pain behind the ear, and diagnosis is based on demonstrating complete facial palsy (i.e., paralysis of both lower face and forehead) in the absence of other neurologic findings. Central lesions that affect fibers before their synapse in the seventh-nerve nucleus in the brainstem spare forehead musculature. In addition to innervating facial musculature, fibers from the seventh nerve innervate the lacrimal gland of the eye (decreasing tearing), the stapedius muscle in the ear (hyperacusis), the submaxillary and sublingual glands, and they carry afferent taste fibers from the anterior two-thirds of the tongue (loss of taste). Most cases are idiopathic (Bell palsy).
Other causes include:

1. Infectious mononucleosis.
2. Lyme disease.
3. Guillain–Barré syndrome (bilateral seventh-nerve palsies, loss of reflexes).
4. Fracture.
5. Severe hypertension.

6. Diabetes.
7. Sarcoid and histiocytosis.
8. An associated otitis or mastoiditis.

Herpes zoster may affect the seventh nerve, causing facial palsy and cutaneous vesicles in the external ear (Ramsay–Hunt syndrome). A cerebellopontine angle tumor or a brainstem plaque from multiple sclerosis may give a peripheral seventh-nerve palsy, usually in association with other cranial nerve signs. Melkersson syndrome is recurrent seventh-nerve palsies associated with facial edema.

Treatment

Treatment with prednisone is commonly used in an attempt to speed recovery. A recent Cochrane review found no evidence to support the efficacy of prednisone in this syndrome. The role of acyclovir in this syndrome is also unclear. An eye shield and methylcellulose eye drops will help prevent corneal ulceration, but patching the eye may cause irritation. Surgical decompression of the facial nerve is probably of no benefit. Patients with hyperacusis, taste loss, or defective tearing have a poorer prognosis (proximal lesion of the facial nerve), as do those with complete (as opposed to partial) facial nerve paralysis. Search specifically for involvement of sixth and fifth cranial nerves, which lie close to the seventh nerve in the brainstem and in the peripheral course of the nerve.

Suggested Readings

Allen D, Dunn L. Aciclovir or valaciclovir for Bell's palsy (idiopathic facial paralysis). *Cochrane Database Syst Rev*. 2004;3: CD001869.

Feinberg JH, Nadler SF, Krivickas LS. Peripheral nerve injuries in the athlete. *Sports Med*. 1997;24:385–408.

Jorns TP, Zakrzewska JM. Evidence-based approach to the medical management of trigeminal neuralgia. *Br J Neurosurg*. 2007;21:253–261.

Lopez BC, Hamlyn PJ, Zakrzewska JM. Systematic review of ablative neurosurgical techniques for the treatment of trigeminal neuralgia. *Neurosurgery*. 2004;54:973–982; discussion 982–983.

Marshall S, Tardif G, Ashworth N. Local corticosteroid injection for carpal tunnel syndrome. *Cochrane Database Syst Rev*. 2007;2:CD001554.

Morgenlander JC, Lynch JR, Sanders DB. Surgical treatment of carpal tunnel syndrome in patients with peripheral neuropathy. *Neurology.* 1997;49:1159–1163.

Nakano KK. Nerve entrapment syndromes. *Curr Opin Rheumatol.* 1997;9:165–173.

Salinas RA, Alvarez G, Ferreira J. Corticosteroids for Bell's palsy (idiopathic facial paralysis). *Cochrane Database Syst Rev.* 2004;4:CD001942.

Muscle Weakness

CASE

A 43-year-old man has a 6-week history of difficulty getting out of bed, arising from a chair, combing his hair, and going up stairs. He has noticed an unusual rash on his knuckles and around his eyelids. He has lost some weight and feels generally fatigued. His examination shows proximal muscle weakness and a rash on his hands and face. His creatine kinase is four times the upper limit of normal.

Diagnosis

Dermatomyositis.

When confronted with a patient who has muscle weakness (Table 11.1), the physician must establish if the weakness is:

1. Myopathic.
2. Due to a neuromuscular junction disorder.
3. More proximal in the nervous system (peripheral nerve, plexus, root, cord, brainstem, brain).

Patients with myopathy tend to have stable weakness. It tends to be proximal, affecting hip and shoulder girdle muscles; except in certain dystrophies, which affect more distal muscles. Patients with neuromuscular junction disorders have proximal muscle weakness that is fatigable, as well as ocular, facial, respiratory, and gustatory muscle weakness. Patients with more proximal problems have the associated features of that neurologic structure (see Chapter 1).

HISTORY

In patients with muscle weakness caused by a *myopathy*, the following occurs:

1. Weakness is usually symmetric and proximal, with the shoulder and pelvic girdle muscles most severely affected. **Climbing stairs, squatting, arising from a chair, and combing the hair are particularly difficult for the myopathic patient.**

■ **TABLE 11.1. Myopathies and Related Disorders**

Acquired myopathies
  Dermatomyositis/polymyositis
  Endocrinopathies
  Steroid-associated
  Alcoholic
  Metabolic
  Inclusion body myositis
Muscular dystrophies
  Duchenne
  Facioscapulohumeral
  Limb-girdle
  Myotonic dystrophy
  Congenital myopathies
Neuromuscular junction disorders
  Myasthenia gravis
  Lambert–Eaton syndrome
  Botulism

2. There are no sensory symptoms (i.e., no "pins-and-needles" sensations or loss of sensation), which are common in neuropathies.
3. Bowel and bladder function are spared.
4. Weakness is usually painless.
5. Cramps may be present, but spasticity is not a feature of the weakness. (Spasticity suggests an upper motor neuron problem.)

In patients with *neuromuscular junction disorders*, the following occurs:

1. Weakness tends to be fluctuating, and worse after exercise or later in the day.
2. Weakness is symmetric and proximal.
3. There may be diplopia, facial muscle weakness, and neck weakness.
4. Swallowing and respiration may be affected.

For myopathies, establish the following points:

1. Is there a *family history* of similar disorders? Muscular dystrophies are often familial.
2. Is there *myotonia* (unable to release grip, slowness to initiate muscle movements)? This suggests one of the myotonic dystrophies.
3. Is there *trouble swallowing*? This is seen frequently in polymyositis.
4. What was the exact *age of onset*? This may help distinguish congenital from acquired myopathies.

For neuromuscular junction disorders, assess whether there is ocular and bulbar weakness, which is common in myasthenia gravis. Is there a dry mouth or bladder symptoms, common in Lambert–Eaton syndrome? Are there prominent autonomic features and a history of tinned food ingestion (botulism)?

PHYSICAL EXAMINATION

Muscle strength can be graded using the MRC scale:

0— no movement.
1—flicker of movement.
2—movement, but not against gravity.
3—movement against gravity, but not resistance.
4—movement against resistance, but not normal strength.
5—normal strength.

In the patient with myopathy:

1. *Proximal limb strength* is more impaired than distal strength except in certain muscular dystrophies. Check deltoids (shoulder), neck flexion, and iliopsoas (hip flexion). Check neck flexion (which is often weaker than neck extension).
2. *Reflexes* are preserved or slightly decreased, except in later stages of muscle weakness.
3. *Sensation* is normal.

In the patient with a neuromuscular junction disorder:

1. Bulbar and neck muscles are commonly affected.
2. Weakness is proximal, but varies.
3. In Eaton–Lambert syndrome, reflexes are reduced before exertion and may increase afterwards. In myasthenia gravis, reflexes tend to be spared.

Check these points, which help to distinguish one cause of muscle weakness from another:

1. Certain muscular dystrophies have a typical pattern. Check for *facial muscle involvement* in facioscapulohumeral dystrophy. Have the patient shut eyes tightly, puff cheeks, or attempt to whistle (difficult in facioscapulohumeral). See if *pelvic and thigh muscles* are most involved, possibly indicating a limb-girdle dystrophy. Check for *myotonia*, by percussing the muscles directly, tapping the tongue, and having the patient close the eyes

tightly to see if the patient has trouble opening them. Patients with myotonia may have trouble "letting go" in a handshake. Such signs are seen in myotonia congenita, myotonic dystrophy, and other myotonic disorders.

2. Check for fatigability and involvement of extraocular muscles, particularly when facial weakness occurs with eyelid ptosis. These are suggestive of neuromuscular junction disorders. Many patients with myasthenia gravis also have dysphagia and dysarthria, and may resort to holding the jaw closed as they eat.

LABORATORY STUDIES

Characteristic features of myopathies include elevated muscle enzymes, especially creatine phosphokinase (CPK) and aldolase, and normal spinal fluid, including CSF protein.

Special studies usually conducted on patients suspected of having myopathies are as follows:

1. *Electromyography* (EMG) and nerve conduction studies. EMG should demonstrate small, polyphasic, early recruiting motor units in the involved muscles consistent with myopathy. Polymyositis may show "irritative features" with fibrillation potentials and high-frequency repetitive discharges. Nerve conduction studies are usually normal.
2. *Muscle biopsy*. Make sure to conduct a biopsy on an affected muscle, and avoid biopsy of a muscle previously used for EMG to avoid artifact from needle insertion.

In neuromuscular junction disorders, repetitive nerve stimulation may show either an incremental or decremental pattern. That is, with repeated stimulation at different rates, the amplitude of the muscle potential may either increase or decrease. This is helpful in showing the presence of neuromuscular junction disorder, and discriminating the different types of NMJ disorders.

IS THERE A TREATABLE MUSCLE WEAKNESS PRESENT?

Check for the following:

1. *Thyroid myopathy*. Myopathy may occur with hyperthyroidism or hypothyroidism. Periodic paralysis is a feature in some patients with Graves disease.

2. *Steroid myopathy*. This commonly occurs in patients taking steroids for other conditions, as well as in Cushing disease. Steroids may exacerbate the myopathy seen in critically ill patients in the intensive care unit (ICU). The CPK is usually normal.

3. *Statin-associated myositis*. Patients taking cholesterol-lowering agents may develop a painful myositis, which improves when the statin is withdrawn.

4. *Dermatomyositis and polymyositis*. There is usually an elevated sedimentation rate, and at times, evidence of other connective tissue disease, such as rheumatoid arthritis or lupus erythematosus. Proximal muscle weakness is typical, and onset is usually subacute. Skin changes with characteristic heliotrope rash are seen with dermatomyositis. Treatment of dermatomyositis and polymyositis includes steroids and immunosuppressant therapy. Approximately 20% of adults with polymyositis have an underlying malignancy.

5. *Inclusion body myositis*. This may be confused with polymyositis. Most patients are middle-aged or elderly men with slowly progressive symmetric weakness. Women are less commonly affected and more likely to be younger. In contrast to other inflammatory myopathies, distal weakness is often as severe as proximal weakness and may include weakness of foot extensors and finger flexors. Pain is uncommon. Most patients have a protracted course that is generally unaffected by immunosuppressive therapies. Muscle biopsy shows typical "inclusion bodies."

6. *Alcoholic myopathy*. These patients may have a subacute and sometimes painful myopathy associated with excessive alcohol ingestion. Does the patient have a concurrent alcoholic cardiac myopathy or neuropathy? Make sure to inquire about alcohol consumption.

7. *Periodic paralysis*. Patients usually have a family history and describe attacks of diffuse muscle weakness lasting hours. Attacks are provoked by cold, food, or exercise. Patients may have a variety of inherited muscle membrane disorders, sometimes characterized by an abnormal potassium level at the time of the attack. Myotonia may be present in the hyperkalemic form.

8. *Myasthenia gravis*. The etiology of myasthenia is an autoimmune attack on acetylcholine receptors of the postsynaptic part of the neuromuscular junction. The patients usually have fluctuating weakness—worse later in the day—often with ptosis, diplopia, and difficulty swallowing. The diagnosis is confirmed with a Tensilon test, repetitive stimulation in a nerve conduction study, single-fiber EMG, and acetylcholine receptor antibody studies. Treatment includes use of anticholinesterases

(e.g., pyridostigmine bromide), steroids, and thymectomy. Sometimes other immunosuppressants, plasmapheresis, or intravenous immunoglobulin are necessary.

9. *Lambert–Eaton syndrome*. This is a rare neuromuscular junction syndrome seen with systemic cancer, especially small-cell cancer of the lung. Proximal weakness and dry mouth are common features. Unlike myasthenia, ocular involvement is rare. Treatment with 4-aminopyridine 3, 4-diaminopyridine, or IVIG has been shown to be effective (level 1B). Removal of the primary tumor may also improve the neuromuscular condition. Repetitive stimulation studies help separate Lambert–Eaton syndrome from myasthenia gravis.

Suggested Readings

Baer AN. Differential diagnosis of idiopathic inflammatory myopathies. *Curr Rheumatol Rep*. 2006;8:178–187.

Cherington M. Botulism: update and review. *Semin Neurol*. 2004;24:155–163.

Dalakas MC. Sporadic inclusion body myositis-diagnosis, pathogenesis, and therapeutic strategies. *Nat Clin Pract Neurol*. 2006;2:437–447.

Maddison P, Newsom-Davis J. Treatment for Lambert-Eaton myasthenic syndrome. *Cochrane Database Syst Rev*. 2005;2: CD003279.

Scherer K, Bedlack RS, Simel DL. Does this patient have myasthenia gravis? *JAMA*. 2005;293:1906–1914.

Skeie GO, Apostolski S, Evoli A. Guidelines for the treatment of autoimmune neuromuscular transmission disorders. *Eur J Neurol* 2006;13:691–699.

12

Tremor and Movement Disorders

CASE

The wife of a 56-year-old man has noticed that he walks behind her when they go to the park. He seems to have problems getting up from chairs and out of bed. When watching television, his left hand shakes. His handwriting has become smaller and difficult to read. He has trouble stepping up on a curb, and sometimes gets stuck in doorways.

Diagnosis

Parkinsonism; probable idiopathic Parkinson disease.

Tremor is a rhythmic oscillating movement of the extremities or head.

Common types of tremor include:

1. Action tremor of the physiologic, essential, or familial type.
2. Intention tremor associated with cerebellar or cerebellar connection disorders.
3. Resting tremor; usually associated with Parkinson disease.

Other movement disorders are discussed in this chapter.

ACTION TREMOR

Action tremor is a tremor that is most prominent when the limb is held out or being used (i.e., with action). Patients notice this tremor when holding a coffee cup, reading the newspaper, writing, or speaking in front of an audience. Action tremor worsens with anxiety or fatigue. Many people have a mild tremor that may be brought out with caffeine, stimulant medications, or theophylline derivatives. This is known as an exaggerated physiologic tremor. Other medications that may cause such a tremor include neuroleptics, tricyclic antidepressants, valproic acid, lithium, and steroids. Hyperthyroidism, pheochromocytoma, hypothermia, and drug and alcohol withdrawal also may cause an exaggerated physiologic tremor. Essential tremor is also an action tremor, but usually of greater amplitude than physiologic tremor. Essential tremors may be seen as a genetically determined trait (familial action tremor). Essential and familial action tremors tend to gradually worsen over years, particularly when patients reach their 60s. One alcoholic drink will decrease action tremors temporarily. In fact, some patients self-medicate with alcohol to their detriment. Aside from the tremor, the neurologic examination is normal in action tremor patients.

Note: **Consider Wilson disease in any young person with an unusual tremor.**

Treatment

Physiologic tremor is treated by removing the cause, if possible (stopping drugs or alcohol, treating medical illness, avoiding caffeine).

The grade A recommendation for essential and familial tremors is to suppress them partially by beta-blockers such as propranolol, or by the use of primidone in small doses (25–500 mg/day, titrated slowly) . Medications that may be useful in a grade B recommendation include topiramate and gabapentin.

INTENTION TREMOR

Intention tremor is not a true tremor, but an impairment of the ability to guide limb movements accurately to their destination. An intention tremor is visible when the patient reaches for an object or the examiner's finger. The patient's arm begins to waver from side to side as it nears its goal, as the brain tries to correct for inaccurate movements. Intention tremor is a useful sign of ataxia. See Chapter 13 for further information on ataxic disorders.

Treatment

There are no well defined treatments for this tremor. Using light weights on the wrists (1 pound) may reduce the tremor amplitude. The long list of medications that have been tried in this condition attests to their limited efficacy.

PARKINSONISM AND REST TREMOR

Parkinsonism refers to a complex of alterations of movement that may be caused by Parkinson disease, or other disorders mimicking Parkinson disease. Features seen in parkinsonism include:

1. Resting tremor.
2. Bradykinesia (decreased movements).

3. Rigidity.
4. Decreased facial expression.
5. Decreased blinking.
6. Shuffling gait.
7. Quiet, hesitant speech pattern (hypophonic).

The resting tremor usually consists of a large amplitude, slow (3–7 Hz), "pill-rolling" tremor that is suppressed with movement, as opposed to action tremors that increase with movement. Often there is small handwriting (micrographia) and postural instability. **The diagnosis of parkinsonism is made by history and clinical exam. There are no diagnostic imaging or laboratory tests.**

The motor manifestations of Parkinson disease are caused by degeneration of dopamine-releasing neurons in the substantia nigra of the midbrain. Cardinal features include tremor, bradykinesia, rigidity, and a gait disorder. Decreased dopamine leads to altered activity in the "extrapyramidal" motor system, which leads to the motor abnormalities described. Parkinson disease is marked pathologically by Lewy bodies and other neuropathologic changes in the remaining neurons of the substantia nigra, and other pigmented nuclei of the brainstem.

Note: **Some patients with Parkinson disease do not have rest tremor (Akinetic-rigid form).**

Not having a rest tremor sometimes concerns clinicians, but this occurs in about 25% of patients with Parkinson disease. Patients with the akinetic-rigid form of Parkinson often have more trouble with gait and rigidity than tremor-predominant patients. If a patient with parkinsonism without tremor doesn't respond to dopamine replacement, he or she may have another form of parkinsonism.

DIFFERENTIAL DIAGNOSIS OF PARKINSONISM

There are other disorders that may cause parkinsonism besides Parkinson disease (sometimes called "Parkinson plus"). These disorders may be difficult to separate clinically from Parkinson disease. A lack of response to medication for Parkinson, early dementia, and other neurologic signs may all suggest such conditions.

Up to 30% of patients with parkinsonism ultimately have a cause other than Parkinson disease.

Consider the following:

1. *Medications* may cause secondary parkinsonism by blocking the D2 receptor in the basal ganglia. Common agents responsible for this effect include typical neuroleptics such as

haloperidol and the anti-emetic metoclopramide. Up to 5% of patients on long-term valproic acid will develop parkinsonism with a cognitive decline that may be reversible.

2. *Progressive supranuclear palsy* (PSP) is a degenerative disorder in which patients have a toppling gait, impaired voluntary up-and-down eye movements, and pseudobulbar palsy. PSP should be considered in a parkinsonian patient who presents with falling as an early symptom.

3. *Multiple system atrophy* (MSA) refers to a group of degenerative disorders in which there are abnormalities in multiple neurologic systems, including the basal ganglia, corticospinal tract, autonomic nervous system, and cerebellum. The Shy–Drager syndrome is a subtype of MSA with impotence, postural hypotension, and parkinsonism. Striatonigral degeneration features parkinsonism and later signs of pyramidal dysfunction, hyperreflexia, extensor toes, and postural instability. Olivopontocerebellar atrophy has prominent brainstem and cerebellar degeneration with associated parkinsonism.

4. *Diffuse Lewy body disease* may cause parkinsonism, accompanied by an early cognitive decline, prominent visual hallucinations, a fluctuating course, and sensitivity to major antipsychotics. Pathologically, Lewy bodies are seen in cortical areas in addition to the pigmented nuclei.

5. *Normal pressure hydrocephalus* (NPH) involves the triad of gait disorder, cognitive decline, and incontinence. Patients may appear parkinsonian but the gait is usually apraxic rather than parkinsonian (patients seem unable to "figure out" how to walk but can still bicycle with their legs effectively when lying in bed on their back). NPH may be a delayed manifestation following a head injury, subarachnoid hemorrhage, meningitis, or may occur spontaneously. On computed tomography (CT) or magnetic resonance imaging, large ventricles are seen without significant atrophy. Gait is "magnetic," with difficulty picking up the feet despite good strength (gait apraxia).

6. Parkinsonism may be secondary to toxins such as chronic manganese or carbon monoxide intoxication.

TREATMENT OF PARKINSON DISEASE

Treatment of Parkinson disease has become a specialized endeavor, with the continuing development of new medications and treatments.

Patients with early Parkinson may not require treatment with medication until they experience difficulty functioning. Selective monoamine oxidase inhibitors, selegiline and rasagiline, may be neuroprotective. To date, unequivocal research support for this theory has been lacking. These have been used as first-line agents in early Parkinson disease. Once difficulty arising from a chair, walking, or using the limbs becomes a problem, medication aimed at improving these functions is indicated.

1. *Levodopa* is the most effective anti-parkinsonian medication, and is the cornerstone of therapy for most patients. Despite this, many physicians delay the use of levodopa until later in the course with the hope that the long-term side effects of this medication can be reduced or delayed. The effect may be dramatic when administered early in disease. Used alone, large doses are needed for effect, and the peripheral effect causes nausea and orthostatic hypotension. When combined with a dopa-decarboxylase inhibitor (carbidopa), the peripheral effects are minimized, and the dose may be reduced as more of the dopa reaches the brain to be converted to dopamine. Combination medication is available as a short-acting or long-acting preparation. The short-acting medication is available as 10/100, 25/100, and 25/250, with the first number referring to the milligrams of carbidopa and the second number referring to the milligrams of levodopa. A long-acting (CR) form is available as 25/100 or 50/200 mg, but does not confer a significant added benefit. Levodopa/carbidopa 25/100, 3 to 4 times a day is the usual starting dose. The most common side effect of levodopa therapy is nausea. Early motor fluctuations, dyskinesia, and on-off phenomena are common problems encountered with levodopa/carbidopa as parkinsonism progresses. Dystonia, agitation, hallucinations, and sleep disorders also may occur, particularly in patients with dementia. Providing levodopa/carbidopa 30 minutes before meals and limiting protein intake during the day may improve absorption and efficacy of levodopa/carbidopa.

2. *Dopamine agonists* are advocated by some authorities as early monotherapy in an attempt to spare the use of levodopa early in the disease. Pergolide, bromocriptine, ropinerole, pramipexole, and rasagiline are available dopamine agonists. Because pergolide, pramipexole, and ropinerole are longer-acting agents, they may help smooth out motor fluctuations seen with levodopa therapy, and have fewer choreiform-like dyskinesias than levodopa. However, they may cause nausea, hypotension, hallucinations, and confusion, as well as excessive somnolence. Gradual titration to the desired dose is the most effective

strategy. They may be used as monotherapy or in combination with other anti-parkinsonian medications.

Ergot derived dopamine agonists (pergolide, bromocryptine, cabergoline) have recently been shown to cause valvular heart disease in up to 5% of treated patients.

In addition, dopamine agonists may cause impulsive behaviors, such as gambling and hypersexuality, particularly at higher doses.

Patients taking dopamine agonists should be warned not to drive if excessive somnolence is a significant complaint. It is not known if lowering the dose of dopamine agonist will help this.

3. *Catecholamine*-O-methyltransferase (COMT) inhibitors (entacapone and tolcopone) extend the pharmacologic half-life of levodopa and may decrease the amount of "off" time.

4. *Selegiline* is a selective monoamine-B oxidase inhibitor that increases the availability of dopamine at the synaptic terminal. A recent Cochrane review indicated that monoamine B inhibitors have an unproven role in early Parkinson disease.

5. *Anticholinergic medications* were used in the past, but are no longer commonly prescribed due to their side effect profile.

6. *Amantidine*, an NMDA antagonist, was initially demonstrated to have a modest anti-parkinsonian effect. This agent is now used to reduce dyskinesias when that side effect of treatment occurs.

7. Small doses of an anti-epileptic medication zonisamide appear to be effective in reducing "off-time" in patients with Parkinson disease (grade B).

8. *Rasagiline*, a selective monoamine-B oxidase inhibitor, was recently approved for use in Parkinson disease. This can be used both as an initial agent early in Parkinson disease, or as an add-on agent for "on-off" problems later in the disease. In the usual dosing of 0.5 to 1.0 mg per day, there do not appear to be problems with reactions to tyramine-containing foods.

There is an increased incidence of melanoma in patients with Parkinson disease. It is unclear if this is related to its treatment or to the disease itself.

TREATMENT OF LATE-STAGE PARKINSON DISEASE

After approximately 5 years of treatment with levodopa, probably because of loss of buffering action by remaining dopaminergic neurons, patients develop a variety of difficult-to-treat side effects of levodopa. Such problems include the following:

1. *Wearing-off* of levodopa may be improved by giving the levodopa more frequently, using longer-acting dopa preparations, adding dopamine agonists to levodopa, adding COMT inhibitors such as tolcapone or entacapone, or adding rasagiline (grade A).

   Fatal hepatotoxicity has occasionally occurred with tolcapone.

2. *Peak-dose dyskinesias.* Use smaller and more frequent levodopa doses, or lower the levodopa dose and add dopamine agonists. Amantidine may also be helpful in this setting.

3. "On-off" fluctuations refer to dramatic, unpredictable shifts from under-treated to over-treated states. These are difficult to treat. Adding dopamine agonists, using COMT inhibitors, using rasagiline, and occasionally using injectable apomorphine may be helpful.

4. Confusion, sleep disorder, and psychosis may be helped by decreasing the medication, particularly limiting anticholinergics, amantidine, and other medications with sedating or anticholinergic effects. Adding clozapine (grade B) or quietipine (grade C) may be used in psychosis. Olanzepine should not be routinely used due to side effects in parkinsonian patients (grade B).

   Clozapine may cause a fatal agranulocytosis and must be closely monitored.

5. Impulse control disorders have recently been identified in patients with Parkinson disease (gambling, hypersexuality, excessive shopping, etc.). These may be associated with the use of dopamine agonists or be related to the disease entity.

6. Deep-brain stimulation of the subthalamic nucleus has been studied in recent randomized trials. These studies showed measurable improvements in activities of daily living, emotional well-being, and mobility, but with a higher risk of serious adverse events including fatal intracerebral hemorrhage (grade B).

OTHER MOVEMENT DISORDERS

1. *Tardive dyskinesia* develops in many patients undergoing prolonged treatment with neuroleptic medications, especially the phenothiazines and haloperidol. These movements may persist long after the drug is withdrawn (tardive). Clinically, patients develop an oral–buccal–lingual dyskinesia with involuntary tongue protrusion, lip smacking, and facial grimacing. Occasional involuntary limb and trunk movements occur. Recent small trials

provide limited data to support specific medications or dose reductions of neuroleptics (grade C). Using atypical antipsychotics may reduce the incidence of this problem.

2. *Hemiballismus* is a wild, flinging movement of an entire limb, caused by disease of the subthalamic nucleus and its connections. It is usually the result of infarction in this area of the brain and may be treated with haloperidol. Untreated, it may cause exhaustion and dehydration.

3. *Acute dystonias* include a variety of abnormal postures, usually with turning of the trunk or limbs in uncomfortable, unnatural directions. These may occur as a side effect of neuroleptic drugs, usually in young adults. Treatment with intravenous diphenhydramine (75 mg) or benztropine mesylate (2 mg) usually will reduce these in minutes. In addition to acute dystonia, tardive dyskinesia, and drug-induced parkinsonism, neuroleptic medications also can cause akathisia, a persistent motor restlessness. Chronic dystonia is caused by a variety of inherited disorders and toxins, as well as idiopathic variants.

4. *Myoclonus*, or jerky, arrhythmic contractions of a muscle or group of muscles, often occurs in a variety of muscle groups (multifocal myoclonus). They occur in a variety of disorders, including anoxia, myoclonic epilepsies, and some degenerative disorders such as Creutzfeldt–Jakob disease. They also can be seen in metabolic encephalopathies (particularly with uremia) and certain drug intoxications (e.g., imipramine toxicity). **Common causes of multifocal myoclonus in hospitalized patients include gabapentin and second- and third-generation cephalosporins, usually in patients with renal insufficiency.** Drugs useful in treatment include clonazepam, valproic acid, and 5-hydroxytryptophan.

5. *Chorea* refers to involuntary, irregular, jerky movements of various body parts, resembling restlessness. Choreic movements are seen in Parkinson disease with dopa therapy, Huntington disease, Sydenham chorea, and lupus erythematosus, in association with pregnancy (chorea gravidarum), and in some children with cerebral palsy. Patients with athetosis have slow writhing movement of the fingers and hands.

6. *Tics* are erratic, coordinated, stereotyped, irresistible behaviors. Some are motor (sudden jerk of the head, shoulder movement, clapping, obscene gestures); whereas others are vocal (snorts, sniffing, occasionally involuntary obscene speech). An obsessive-compulsive disorder often coexists with the tics. Tics may develop as part of a symptom complex in Gilles de la Tourette syndrome.

Suggested Readings

Deane KH, Spieker S, Clarke CE. Catechol-O-methyltransferase inhibitors for levodopa-induced complications in Parkinson's disease. *Cochrane Database Syst Rev*. 2004;4:CD004554.

Deuschl G, Schade-Brittinger C, Krack P, et al. A randomized trial of deep-brain stimulation for Parkinson's disease. *N Engl J Med*. 2006;355:896–908.

Lewis ED. Essential tremor. *Clin Geriatr Med*. 2006;22:843–857.

Macleod AD, Counsell CE, Ives N, et al. Monoamine oxidase B inhibitors for early Parkinson's disease. *Cochrane Database of Syst Rev*. 2007; 4. John Wiley & Sons, Ltd. DOI: 10.1002/14651858. CD004898.pub2.

Murata M, Hasegawa K, Kanazawa I. Zonisamide improves motor function in Parkinson disease: a randomized, double-blind study. *Neurology*. 2007;68:45–50.

Ristic AJ, Vojvodic N, Jankovic S, et al. The frequency of reversible parkinsonism and cognitive decline associated with valproate treatment. *Epilepsia*. 2006;47:2183–2185.

Soares-Weiser K, Rathbone J. Neuroleptic reduction and/or cessation and neuroleptics as specific treatments for tardive dyskinesia. *Cochrane Database Syst Rev*. 2006;1:CD000459.

Watts RL, Killer WC. *Movement Disorders, Neurologic Principles and Practice*. 2nd ed. New York: McGraw-Hill; 2004.

Weisman D, McKeith I. Dementia with lewy bodies. *Semin Neurol*. 2006;27:42–47.

Zanettini R, Antonini A, Gatto G, et al. Valvular heart disease and the use of dopamine agonists for Parkinson's disease. *N Engl J Med*. 2007;356:39–46.

Ataxia

CASE

A 34-year-old obese female undergoes gastric bypass surgery. She loses 75 pounds in 2 months, and develops acutely unsteady gait with nystagmus on lateral gaze, and confusion. Thiamine is given IV in the emergency room. She returns to normal after 1 week.

Diagnosis

Wernicke encephalopathy, due to thiamine deficiency from malabsorption.

Ataxia is a disorder of coordination and rhythm. With ataxia, the rate, range, and force of movement are altered. Classically, physicians are taught that ataxia is equivalent to a cerebellar disorder. Indeed, this may be so. However since the advent of more advanced imaging, it has become clear that many people with ataxia actually have disorders in other parts of the systems that underlie movement.

Remember, ataxia does not always equal "cerebellar." Signs of ataxia include the following:

1. Intention tremor that with voluntary movement of a limb towards a target, sees side-to-side oscillation, which increases as the limb closes in on the target.
2. Unsteady gait, often with a wide base.
3. Dysdiadochokinesis, where when alternately supinating and pronating the hand, there are slow, jerky, arrhythmic movements.
4. Overshoot dysmetria, where the patient often launches a limb to the target, overshoots, and then recorrects. This is the basis of intention tremor.
5. Scanning speech, in which ataxia is sometimes associated with a hesitant, arrhythmic speech that varies in rate and force.

IS THE LESION IN THE FRONTAL LOBE?

Mechanism: involvement of corticocerebellar connections (i.e., frontopontocerebellar pathway).

1. *Tumor*. Meningioma, glioma, or metastatic tumor may involve the frontal lobes. Patients may have signs suggesting cerebellar disease (i.e., staggering gait, difficulty performing rapid alternating movements, and even nystagmus). Patients with "frontal ataxia" tend to fall backward. Other features of frontal lobe dysfunction include perseveration, grasp and primitive suck reflexes, incontinence, slowness in thinking and initiating conversation, and headache.
2. *Anterior cerebral artery syndrome*. A thrombotic occlusion of this artery affects the frontal lobes (see Chapter 16). A large aneurysm of the anterior communicating artery also may affect the frontal lobes.
3. *Hydrocephalus*. Enlargement of the frontal horns of the lateral ventricles affects leg fibers, and may produce ataxia. In addition, there are often memory loss and incontinence. Hydrocephalus may occur with tumors that obstruct the ventricular system, or with disorders of cerebrospinal fluid (CSF) absorption (see Chapter 31).

IS THE LESION SUBCORTICAL?

Mechanism: involvement of corticocerebellar connections, plus pyramidal tract dysfunction.

1. *Multiple strokes* (état lacunaire). In addition to ataxia, there is emotional lability, brisk reflexes including increased jaw jerk, dysarthria, and dementia (see Chapter 19).
2. *Ataxic hemiparesis* (ataxia crural paresis). This is a lacunar syndrome, with the lesion in the internal capsule or contralateral basis pontis. There is ataxia on the same side as the hemiparesis, with weakness primarily in the leg.

IS THE LESION IN THE THALAMUS?

Mechanism: involvement of ventral lateral (VL) nucleus and adjacent subthalamic region.

Occasionally, patients with thalamic infarction may develop a sensory ataxia, with noncoordination based on a profound loss of position sense. This will be unilateral, affecting arm and leg. Check for sensory loss in any patient with ataxia. Lesions in the denta-torubrothalamic projection to the VL nucleus of the thalamus result in hemiataxia of the contralateral limbs.

IS THE LESION IN THE BRAINSTEM?

Mechanism: involvement of cerebellar connections.

The two most common causes of ataxia, secondary to brain-stem lesions are stroke and multiple sclerosis. Diagnosis is based on history and findings of other brainstem signs (e.g., crossed motor or sensory findings, internuclear ophthalmoplegia, nystag-mus, dysarthria).

IS THE LESION IN THE CEREBELLUM?

Mechanism: direct involvement of coordination pathways.

1. *Signs*. Signs of cerebellar dysfunction include limb, trunk, gait, and speech ataxia, nystagmus, and hypotonia. Depending on whether midline or lateral cerebellar structures are involved, there may or may not be limb ataxia or prominent gaze-evoked nystagmus. Midline cerebellar lesions produce truncal and gait ataxia. **Cerebellar hemisphere lesions characteristically cause ipsilateral limb ataxia and nystagmus.** An impaired checking response (unable to halt sudden movements) may be present. A subtle cerebellar disorder may be detected by problems with tandem gait (walking with one foot in front of the other). Scanning speech is characteristic of cerebellar ataxia.
   Note: Cerebellar hemispheric lesions cause ipsilateral ataxia.
2. *Cerebellar hemorrhage, infarction, tumor.* These may have occip-ital headache and ocular gaze palsies. Limb strength and sensa-tion are often preserved. Symptoms may be limited to headache and difficulty walking. *Remember the need for emer-gency computed tomography scan for diagnosis, and often the need for surgical intervention* (see Chapter 16). Primary cerebellar tumors are seen in childhood; they are rare in adults. Metastatic tumors often involve the cerebellum in adults.
3. *Spinocerebellar degenerations.* These syndromes include olivo-pontocerebellar degeneration and Friedreich ataxia, among others. In Friedreich ataxia, there is usually a positive family history, a chronic course, and evidence of more widespread nervous system involvement such as peripheral neuropathy (loss of reflexes) and pyramidal tract dysfunction (upgoing toes). Pes cavus (high arched feet) or scoliosis sometimes is associated with

these degenerations. The genetics of the spinocerebellar degenerations is now better understood and there are genetic tests for
some of the forms of spinocerebellar disease.

4. *Alcoholism* or occult malignancy. These may be associated with
cerebellar degeneration. Alcoholic cerebellar degeneration is
characterized by ataxia of gait and of the legs, with less prominent involvement of arms, speech, or ocular motility. There is
usually an associated memory loss and polyneuropathy. Acute
ataxia, confusion, and oculomotor paralysis associated with
alcoholism or nutritional deficits (Wernicke encephalopathy)
responds to thiamine administration (see Chapter 27).

5. *Occult malignancy*. Subacute cerebellar ataxia may be a presenting symptom of occult malignancy, especially carcinoma of
the breast or ovary. Check for anti-Yo antibodies in serum or
CSF.

6. *Acute cerebellitis*. This is a viral or post-viral cause of ataxia seen
in children and rarely in adults.

7. Recently a syndrome of progressive ataxia has been described
in carriers of the fragile X. Other features include essential
tremor, dementia, and neuropsychiatric syndromes. This condition should be considered whenever there is progressive
ataxia or tremor and a family history of mental retardation.

IS THE LESION IN THE SPINAL CORD?

Mechanism: ataxia through posterior column dysfunction,
involvement of pyramidal tracts. Remember, a positive Romberg
sign (unsteady stance with eyes closed, steady with eyes open)
usually indicates posterior column disease. Magnetic resonance
imaging (MRI) is usually diagnostic.

1. Patients with *cervical spondylosis* with associated cervical
myelopathy usually have neck and arm pain and abnormal cervical spine films. Depending on the extent of spinal cord
involvement, there may be posterior column dysfunction and
upgoing toes due to pyramidal tract involvement.

2. *Multiple sclerosis* often involves the spinal cord. Diagnosis is
made on the basis of finding multiple lesions of the nervous
system (e.g., optic neuritis, brainstem signs), a history of attacks
separated in time, elevation of CSF gamma globulin, and an
abnormal brain MRI.

3. *Vitamin B_{12} deficiency* may produce subacute combined
degeneration, with involvement of the lateral and posterior
columns of the spinal cord. Ataxia is based on a combination of

weakness and position sense loss. Often there is also a peripheral neuropathy making the interpretation of physical signs more difficult.

4. Other causes of ataxia secondary to spinal cord dysfunction include spinal cord tumor and tabes dorsalis.

IS THE LESION IN THE PERIPHERAL NERVE?

Mechanism: ataxia secondary to weakness or loss of position sense.

1. *Miller–Fisher syndrome* is an acute syndrome characterized by ataxia, loss of deep tendon reflexes, and ophthalmoparesis. It is considered a variant of Guillain–Barré syndrome.
2. Ataxia also may be a feature of several *peripheral neuropathies* from other causes (sensory ataxia). Some patients develop a sensory ataxia from degeneration of the dorsal root ganglia, a ganglioneuritis. This can be seen with remote neoplasms (paraneoplastic neuropathy), Sjögren syndrome, chemotherapy, or as an idiopathic disorder.
3. Occasionally, early in Guillain–Barré syndrome, gait ataxia may precede frank muscle weakness and reflex loss.

Suggested Readings

Bolla L, Palmer RM. Paraneoplastic cerebellar degeneration. Case report and literature review. *Arch Intern Med.* 1997;157: 1258–1262.

Fogel BL, Perlman S. Clinical features and molecular genetics of autosomal recessive cerebellar ataxias. *Lancet Neurol.* 2007;6: 245–257.

Hainline B, Tuszynski MH, Posner JB. Ataxia in epidural spinal cord compression. *Neurology.* 1992;42:2193–2195.

Koeppen AH. The hereditary ataxias. *J Neuropathol Exp Neurol.* 1998:57:531–543.

Lapergue B, Klein I, Olivot JM, et al. Diffusion weighted imaging of cerebellar lesions in Wernicke's encephalopathy. *J Neuroradiol.* 2006;33:126–128.

Melo TP, Bogousslavsky J, Mouline T, et al. Thalamic ataxia. *J Neurol.* 1992;239:1432–1459.

Paulson H, Ammache Z. Ataxia and hereditary disorders. *Neurol Clin.* 2001;19:759–782.

Terry JB, Rosenberg RN. Frontal lobe ataxia. *Surg Neurol.* 1995;44:583–588.

14

Sleep Disorders

CASE

A 45-year-old electrician comes to you for his "epilepsy." He has been treated for years by another neurologist with up to three anti-epileptic drugs at a time without success. He has episodes where he feels "goofed up" and may lose awareness. Friends note that he "just lies there" for a few minutes then comes around. Sometimes he feels weak when he hears a funny joke. He used to fall asleep during high school classes.

Diagnosis

Narcolepsy with cataplexy.

Sleep disorders are more common than generally realized. Approximately 10% to 15% of the population has sleep-related problems. Early diagnosis and proper treatment depend on an awareness of characteristic symptoms.

Sleep disorders are separated into three groups:

1. Disorders of excessive somnolence (DOES), such as narcolepsy and sleep apnea.
2. Disorders of initiation and maintenance of sleep (DIMS), such as insomnia.
3. Abnormal behaviors caused by sleep disorders (parasomnias), such as sleepwalking and night terrors.

Take a sleep history from the patient *and* the bed partner:

1. When does the patient go to bed? How long until the patient falls asleep? Does the patient wake up at night? When does the patient awaken in the morning?
2. What medications or stimulants does the patient take? What beverages does the patient drink? What activities are done before going to bed?
3. Does the patient toss and turn (unrestorative sleep)? Are there sudden jerking leg movements ("periodic leg movements")?
4. Does the patient feel the urge to move the legs from time to time (restless leg syndrome)? Is there loud snoring, or are there long pauses between breaths (sleep apnea)?

5. Does the patient have unusual activities at night, such as sleep-walking, or violent dreams (parasomnias)? Do they act out dreams, thrashing around in bed (REM behavior disorder)?
6. Does the patient wake up feeling refreshed, even after a short nap (narcolepsy)?

The examination is usually not helpful in the diagnosis of sleep disorders.

DISORDERS OF EXCESSIVE SOMNOLENCE (DOES)

Manifestations of excessive sleepiness or drowsiness during the day; including falling asleep during activities such as eating, driving, or sitting in a class. The causes include situational sleep deprivation (e.g., students who stay awake too late, parents with small children), use of certain medications or intoxicants (e.g., sedatives, antidepressants, muscle relaxants, ethanol), depression (may decrease or increase sleep time), or disorders of sleep such as narcolepsy or sleep apnea.

NARCOLEPSY

In narcolepsy, a genetically determined disorder, patients have one or more of the following:

1. *Sleep attacks*, which are uncontrollable attacks of sleep for short periods.
2. *Cataplexy*, consisting of sudden loss of muscle tone, induced by emotion or sudden stimuli.
3. *Sleep paralysis*, in which upon waking or in transition to sleep, the patient is unable to move.
4. *Hypnagogic hallucinations*, including vivid dreamlike hallucinations just before falling asleep or when just awakening.
5. *Automatic behavior*, which is attention lapses in which routine activities are continued, and the patient is amnesic for the behavior.

SLEEP APNEA

In sleep apnea, the patient may have one or more of the following: heavy snoring, apneic episodes during sleep, restless sleep, morning headaches, memory disturbances, learning problems, and hypertension. Seizure disorders and headache disorders may be worsened by sleep apnea.

1. *Obstructive sleep apnea* is a condition in which patients have respiratory movements in sleep, but excessive weight, or an abnormal oropharynx make these ineffective. The consequence is snoring and episodes of breathing cessation. Oxygenation decreases during the episodes, and sleep is often disrupted and of poor quality. Hypertension, polycythemia, arrhythmias, and cor pulmonale may occur if sleep apnea is untreated.

2. *Central sleep apnea* has been observed with a variety of neurologic disorders that disrupt the lower brainstem. Here, episodes of apnea are unaccompanied by respiratory movements. Central sleep apnea is much less common than obstructive sleep apnea. Patients may have a combination of obstructive and central sleep apnea.

DISORDERS OF INITIATION AND MAINTENANCE OF SLEEP (DIMS)

The patient with insomnia cannot fall asleep at night, has difficulty staying asleep, and/or wakes up early. Disturbed nocturnal sleep leads to daytime drowsiness. Consider the following:

1. Does the patient participate in stimulating activities before sleep, such as exercising, paying the bills, or in many instances, watching television?

2. Are there symptoms of depression, including poor appetite, early awakening, weight loss, or sadness?

3. Does the patient have chronic renal failure or alcoholism, each of which has been associated with secondary sleep disorders?

4. Does the patient take certain medications, such as caffeine, stimulants, and certain antidepressants, which may cause secondary insomnia?

PARASOMNIAS

In parasomnias, abnormal behaviors occur in association with sleep.

1. *Sleepwalking* is common, usually is seen in childhood, and may suggest a psychiatric disorder or medication intoxication if it begins in adulthood.

2. *Body jerks and sensory symptoms* while falling asleep are common and usually benign.

3. *Paroxysmal bursts* of choreoathetoid movements in sleep (*nocturnal paroxysmal dystonia*) may respond to antiepileptic drugs.

4. *Night terrors* are common in childhood. Children awaken with fright, tachycardia, and inconsolable distress for a few minutes. Children tend to outgrow this condition. **Night terrors are a common cause of neurologic consultation for normal children.**

5. *Violent behavior* in rapid eye movement (REM) sleep may occur in older males, and may be dangerous to the patient and bed partner if left untreated. Many of these patients later develop parkinsonism (Parkinson disease or Lewy Body disease).

6. Seizures may occur in sleep, and may be difficult to separate from non-epileptic parasomnias.

7. Restless leg syndrome (RLS). This is a common parasomnia that may disrupt sleep. Patients with this problem experience a sensation of "having to move the legs" at bedtime. This can be very irritating and may cause them to have to get up repeatedly during the night. Elderly patients, and patients with renal failure, Parkinson disease, iron deficiency anemia, and people with multiple sclerosis are more prone to RLS.

LABORATORY EVALUATION

In narcolepsy, the results of a sleep electroencephalogram (EEG) combined with electromyographic (EMG) and electrooculographic monitoring (a polysomnogram) are frequently abnormal, showing REM sleep at sleep outset rather than later in the sleep cycle. Results of a multiple sleep latency test, which measures the time to fall asleep (latency), are usually abnormal. In sleep apnea, a record of the patient's breathing pattern during sleep is necessary. Monitoring O_2, respiratory efforts, and electrocardiogram can help distinguish between obstructive, central, or mixed types of sleep apnea. Periodic leg movements can be recorded by monitoring EMG activity of the legs during sleep. Parasomnias are recorded by a combination of EEG and video monitoring in the setting of a sleep study. These studies are best performed in laboratories with a particular interest and expertise in sleep disorders.

TREATMENT

1. *Sleep apnea:* Continuous positive airway pressure at night may prove helpful in treatment, and reduces awakenings and daytime sleepiness. Stimulants and rarely diaphragmatic pacing are used in the central type. There is no good randomized trial evidence for effective medications in obstructive sleep apnea.

2. *Narcolepsy:* Frequent naps and judicious use of stimulant drugs, such as methylphenidate, are helpful in narcolepsy. Modafinil is chemically distinct from stimulant drugs and is FDA approved in narcolepsy. Tricyclic antidepressants, such as protriptyline and clomipramine, are useful in cataplexy. Sodium oxybate was recently approved by the FDA for a small group of patients with cataplexy and narcolepsy; there are safety and abuse concerns about this medicine that limit its use.

3. *Insomnia:* The treatment of insomnia is difficult and must be tailored to the individual patient. Modalities include environmental manipulation (e.g., altering bedtime routine, doing a relaxing evening exercise, taking a hot bath before sleep), relaxation techniques, psychotherapy, and short-term hypnotic drug use. Remember, elderly patients normally require less sleep than when they were younger.

   Useful tips for patients with insomnia:

   - Reserve bed for sleeping and sex (i.e., no eating, reading, watching television, or tossing and turning).
   - Go to sleep at the same time every night, and get up at the same time every morning.
   - Do not eat large meals before bed.
   - Do not consume alcohol as a hypnotic.
   - If unable to sleep after a fixed amount of time (e.g., 40 minutes), get up and do something else.
   - Turn the clock around so you cannot see it; there is no value in being aware of how late it is when you cannot sleep.

4. *Restless leg syndrome:* Ropinarole is the first FDA-approved medication for use in restless leg syndrome. A regular exercise program improves restless leg syndrome (level 1b).

5. *REM behavior disorder:* Clonazepam is usually efficacious for this condition. Patients with REM behavior disorder should be observed for the development of parkinsonian syndromes, which are commonly related to this sleep disorder.

Suggested Readings

Aukerman MM, Aukerman D, Bayard M, et al. Exercise and restless legs syndrome: a randomized controlled trial. *J Am Board Fam Med*. 2006;19:487–493.

Barthlen GM. Sleep disorders. Obstructive sleep apnea, restless legs syndrome, and insomnia in geriatric patients. *Geriatrics*. 2002; 57:34–39.

Gagnon JF, Postuma RB, Montplaisir J. Update on the pharmacology of REM sleep behavior disorder. *Neurology*. 2006;67:742–747.

Montplaisir J, Karrasch J, Haan J, et al. Ropinirole is effective in the long-term management of restless legs syndrome: a randomized controlled trial. *Mov Disord*. 2006;21:1627–1635.

Smith I, Lasserson TJ, Wright J. Drug therapy for obstructive sleep apnoea in adults. *Cochrane Database Syst Rev*. 2006;2:CD003002.

Thorpy M. Therapeutic advances in narcolepsy. *Sleep Med*. 2007;8: 427–440.

Wolkove N, Elkholy O, Baltzan M, et al. Sleep and aging: 1. Sleep disorders commonly found in older people. *CMAJ*. 2007;176: 1299–1304.

15

Stroke

CASE

A 67-year-old man with diabetes, long-standing hypertension, and a pack-a-day smoking habit presents to the emergency room 45 minutes after suddenly dropping his fork from his right hand at lunch. In the emergency room, he shows signs of a global aphasia, right hemiparesis affecting the arm and face more than the leg, and moderate hypertension. A CT scan is negative. He is considered for thrombolytic therapy.

Diagnosis

Cerebral infarction in left hemisphere, caused by embolus or thrombosis in the middle cerebral artery territory.

Stroke is one of the most common neurologic problems. It is the third leading cause of death in the United States. This chapter presents a basic approach to the patient with stroke, and outlines generally accepted therapy. Therapy of stroke is evolving with the introduction of newer medications and interventions.

STROKE TYPES

Stroke is a general term for the sudden onset of a focal neurologic deficit caused by vascular disease. There are subcategories of stroke, each with a specific cause, course, and treatment (Table 15.1). Infarction refers to stroke in which there is a loss of blood supply to part of the brain, so that ischemic injury occurs in one part of the brain. Infarction may be thrombotic (i.e., caused by blood clot formation within a vessel) or embolic (caused by material formed proximally, such as at a heart valve or carotid plaque, and then dislodged to occlude a distal vessel). Thrombotic stroke is often characterized as large vessel (e.g., carotid, vertebral, or basilar arteries) or small vessel (e.g., the lenticulostriate branches of the middle cerebral artery). Cerebral hemorrhage refers to abnormal bleeding within the skull. This may be intracerebral (in the brain parenchyma) or surrounding the brain (subarachnoid, subdural, or epidural).

■ TABLE 15.1. Stroke Types
Infarction
Thrombotic
Large vessel
Small vessel
Embolic
Hemorrhage
Intracerebral
Deep
Lobar
Subarachnoid
Epidural
Subdural

WHERE IS THE STROKE? WHAT IS THE ANATOMY?

1. Intracerebral hemorrhage is usually deep in the brain, and may affect the putamen, thalamus, cerebellum, or pons. Lobar hemorrhages also occur.
2. Emboli tend to produce superficial wedge-shaped infarcts as a result of the distal migration of emboli, giving cortical deficits or deficits at the top of the basilar artery territory.
3. Thrombosis produces a variety of syndromes with the diagnosis based on history, anatomy of the lesion, mechanism of the thrombosis, and exclusion of embolic or hemorrhagic strokes. Any part of the brain or brainstem may be involved in thrombotic stroke.
4. Lacunar strokes usually involve the deep white matter, basal ganglia, or brainstem. The small, well-circumscribed lesions of lacunar disease cause characteristic clinical symptoms and signs that strongly suggest the diagnosis of lacunar disease (see Chapter 16).
5. Subarachnoid hemorrhage causes sudden and severe headache and stiff neck, and may also cause symptoms at the hemorrhage site (e.g., anterior communicating artery: mutism and paraparesis). Often there is no focal neurologic deficit.

HOW DID THE STROKE DEVELOP?

1. Intracranial hemorrhage occurs during waking hours, usually in a known hypertensive patient, or in a patient with a bleeding tendency (e.g., a patient receiving anticoagulant medication).

The full deficit is seldom present at onset but develops gradually over minutes to hours. There is usually no warning prior to the acute bleed. Headache, nausea, and vomiting are usually, but not invariably, present.

2. Emboli usually give a maximal deficit at onset, and often occur during waking hours. The deficit may improve in hours. There may be headache or focal seizures.

3. Thrombosis often occurs during sleep or is present on awakening. Symptoms and signs usually progress in a stepwise fashion; it may take hours or days for the full deficit to develop. A warning is common in thrombotic strokes. The patient may have a headache and frequently has a history of prior transient ischemic attacks (TIAs), which are brief episodes of neurologic symptoms resulting from vascular disease (see Chapter 17).

4. Lacunar or small-vessel thrombotic strokes occur either abruptly or in a stuttering course over hours or days. There may be warning TIAs, but headache is uncommon. There are usually risk factors such as hypertension, hyperlipidemia, smoking, and diabetes.

5. Subarachnoid hemorrhage occurs abruptly with a severe, "worst headache of my life" as the cardinal feature. Onset may be during exertion, with an associated stiff neck and photophobia. A "sentinel" headache may occur days or weeks prior to a major subarachnoid hemorrhage.

WHAT ARE HISTORICAL CLUES AND PHYSICAL FINDINGS?

Is there evidence for occlusion or stenosis of the internal or common carotid artery?

1. One of the most common causes of TIA or stroke is atherosclerotic disease affecting the internal carotid artery at its origin, with stroke occurring as a result of thrombosis of the vessel or embolism to distal branches of the internal carotid.

2. Clinical signs may include a carotid bruit (most significant if high pitched, and at the angle of the jaw), contralateral ocular bruit, or a decreased pulsation of the carotid in the neck. Horner syndrome may be seen ipsilateral to a carotid occlusion or dissection.

   The presence of a carotid bruit does not reliably predict severe carotid stenosis, and the absence of a carotid bruit does not rule out severe carotid stenosis (poor test sensitivity and specificity). Imaging studies need to be done that reliably measure the carotid (e.g., carotid ultrasound, angiogram).

■ **TABLE 15.2. Major Cerebrovascular Disorders that Cause Stroke**

Infarction
  Atherosclerosis /thrombosis
  Embolism
  Fibromuscular dysplasia
  Hypercoagulable states
  Dissection
  Vasculitis
  Sickle-cell anemia
  Drug use
  Inherited (e.g., cadasil, MELAS, Fabry)
Hemorrhage
  Hypertensive hemorrhage
  Congophilic angiopathy
  Aneurysm rupture
  AVM
  Trauma
  Bleeding disorders (e.g., hemophilia, anticoagulants)

3. Occasionally, atheromatous emboli (Hollenhorst plaques) to the retinal arteries may be seen on funduscopic examination on the same side as a carotid stenosis.
4. Noninvasive testing including duplex carotid ultrasound, and transcranial Doppler (TCD) help identify and characterize carotid lesions. Each of these tests assesses different aspects of cerebrovascular flow and anatomy, and may be used to determine the degree of stenosis and abnormalities of carotid flow (Table 15.2). Magnetic resonance angiography (MRA) may also be useful in assessing carotid stenosis. A combination of noninvasive vascular testing and imaging is supplanting conventional angiography in preoperative assessment for carotid endarterectomy. CT angiography (CTa) is another technique that is useful in showing stenosis in extracranial and intracranial vessels, but carries a large radiation load and moderate IV dye load.

LARGE-VESSEL OR SMALL-VESSEL DISEASE?

Warning symptoms tend to be stereotyped in small-vessel disease and occur over hours to days. In large-vessel disease, the symptoms frequently vary depending on which territory of the vessel is involved during the warning; symptoms usually precede the stroke by days or weeks, but may occur over a period of months. See Table 15.2 for cerebrovascular diseases that cause stroke.

Headache is common with large-vessel occlusion. Posterior circulation stroke often produces headache over the occiput, and anterior circulation stroke usually produces headache behind the eyes or over the forehead or temples. Headache rarely accompanies small-vessel occlusion.

IS THERE AN EMBOLIC FOCUS?

The heart is the most common source of emboli, although emboli may arise from a plaque in a diseased carotid artery or aorta. Cardiogenic emboli account for 15% to 20% of all ischemic strokes. Cardiac factors predisposing to emboli include:

1. Mural thrombi, especially with anterior wall myocardial infarction (MI) and left-ventricular wall abnormality (emboli usually occur within 10 days but sometimes months after the MI and may be the presenting feature of an MI).
2. Mitral valve disease.
3. Atrial fibrillation.

Transesophageal echocardiography is valuable in more clearly imaging cardiac abnormalities that serve as potential sources of stroke. These include:

1. Mural thrombus.
2. Atrial septal defects.
3. Atrial septal aneurysms.
4. Patent foramen ovale.
5. Atherosclerotic plaques in the ascending aorta.

Paroxysmal cardiac arrhythmias are an important cause of embolic stroke, and may require a Holter monitor for detection. Atrial fibrillation is a major independent risk factor for stroke, whether persistent or paroxysmal. Other cardiac embolic risk factors include prosthetic or calcified valves, bacterial endocarditis, marantic endocarditis, atrial myxoma, and non-ischemic cardiomyopathies.

IS THERE A COAGULATION DEFICIT OR SYSTEMIC CAUSE OF STROKE?

Stroke may occur in the absence of vascular disease, cardiac source, or trauma. In such cases, a coagulation deficit may be the underlying mechanism. Hypercoagulable states may occur during surgery, infection, or pregnancy. A variety of familial coagulation deficits that predispose to thrombosis are known, such as protein C and S deficiencies, antithrombin III deficiency, sickle-cell anemia, factor V Leiden, and the prothrombin gene mutation. The lupus anticoagulant and antiphospholipid antibodies may be important risk factors in strokes in the young. Drug and alcohol abuse is associated with a variety of strokes, both thrombotic and hemorrhagic.

IS THERE AN INTRACRANIAL HEMORRHAGE?

1. The diagnosis of subarachnoid hemorrhage (SAH) is usually apparent from the history and physical examination. A non-contrast CT scan is often diagnostic, but in approximately 5% of cases the CT is negative. In such cases, a lumbar puncture is important because it may show bloody cerebrospinal fluid (CSF), elevated pressure, increased protein, or xanthochromia (a yellowish tinge of the CSF caused by red blood cell break-down). If subarachnoid hemorrhage has occurred, four-vessel angiography will help in locating the source of bleeding; most typically from an intracranial berry aneurysm (approximately 20% of such aneurysms are multiple). A CTa or MRA can identify larger aneurysms, but neither is the "gold-standard" for diagnosis. In patients with a subarachnoid bleed and a negative angiogram, magnetic resonance imaging (MRI) may show thrombus inside an aneurysm, avoiding misdiagnosis. With MRI-negative SAH, a repeat cerebral angiogram is often recommended a few days or weeks after the initial scan to rule out occult aneurysms.

2. Intracerebral hemorrhage is usually evident on the CT or MRI scan, and is suspected clinically by progressive deficit over hours or minutes, and the presence of decreased consciousness, both of which are common in this disorder. The most common causes of nontraumatic intracerebral hemorrhage are hypertension and trauma. Other causes include:

   Blood dyscrasias.
   Anticoagulants.
   Drug abuse (cocaine or amphetamines).
   Amyloid angiopathy.
   Brain tumors.
   Arteriovenous malformations (AVMs).

   Amyloid angiopathy: a condition in elderly patients where blood vessels in the brain spontaneously rupture due to deposition of

■ **TABLE 15.3. Characteristic Features of Stroke**

	Embolus	Large-Vessel Thrombosis	Small-Vessel Thrombosis	Hemorrhage
Location	Cortical wedge	Variable	Basal ganglia, capsule, pons	Deep or lobar
Onset	Sudden	Sudden or stepwise	Sudden or stepwise	Progressive over minutes, hours
Warning?	Usually no	May have TIA	May have TIA	No
Headache?	Sometimes	Sometimes	No	Usually
CT scan	Decreased density[a]	Decreased density[a]	Small decreased density	Increased density, mass effect, edema
MRI	High signal DWI early	High signal DWI early	High signal DWI early	Variable depending on duration of hemorrhage

[a]May not be visible until 12 to 24 hours after acute onset with infarction of either embolic or thrombotic type. May be accompanied by dense MCA sign with thrombus visible in the middle cerebral artery on CT.

amyloid material in the vessel walls. Often associated with Alzheimer disease.

See Table 15.3 for characteristic features of stroke.

STROKE IN YOUNG ADULTS

When evaluating stroke in young adults, pursue risk factors such as use of oral contraceptives, previously undetected hypertension, mitral valve prolapse, patent foramen ovale with paradoxical embolism, hypercoagulable states, and metabolic disorders (e.g., homocystinuria).

Cocaine abuse, binge or high alcohol consumption, and smoking are important causes of stroke in the young adult. Stroke syndromes associated with cocaine include:

1. Subarachnoid hemorrhage caused by rupture of aneurysms and AVMs.
2. Intracerebral hemorrhage.
3. Cerebral infarction.

Excessive alcohol consumption is associated with hypertension, intracranial hemorrhage, cerebral infarction, and increased risk of death from stroke. Abuse of amphetamine has been associated with intracranial hemorrhage ("speed" hemorrhage).

Arterial dissection is an important cause of stroke in young adults and often is heralded by sharp pain in the neck. With carotid dissection, patients often have a Horner syndrome due to sympathetic involvement in the carotid sheath. Dissection may result from trauma, neck exercise, or cervical manipulation, although it is often spontaneous. Some patients have redundant loops in the carotid arteries. Imaging with MRA or CTa is usually diagnostic.

LABORATORY INVESTIGATION

Laboratory investigation of the stroke patient should include the following:

- *Complete blood count:* blood dyscrasia, polycythemia, thrombocytopenia, thrombocytosis, or infection (neutrophilia) as risk factors for stroke.
- *Prothrombin time, partial thromboplastin time:* clue to the patient with antiphospholipid antibody (prolonged partial thromboplastin time), or other coagulopathy.
- *Urinalysis:* hematuria in subacute bacterial endocarditis (SBE), with embolic stroke.
- *Sedimentation rate:* elevation a clue to vasculitis, hyperviscosity, or SBE as cause of stroke.
- *Chest radiograph:* enlarged heart as embolic source of stroke, or evidence of prolonged hypertension; may detect an unsuspected malignancy.
- *Electrocardiogram:* may reveal arrhythmia, recent myocardial infarct, or enlarged left atrium as a source of embolism.
- *Risk factor screen:* lipid profile, hemoglobin A1c, homocysteine. Consider the evaluation of thrombotic risk factors; usually included in a thrombotic risk panel (e.g., anti-phospholipid antibodies, protein C, S).

CRANIAL COMPUTERIZED TOMOGRAPHY

The CT scan is useful in separating hemorrhagic (intracerebral or subarachnoid hemorrhage) from non-hemorrhagic (thrombotic or embolic) stroke. Blood present in a fresh hemorrhage produces an area of increased density; infarction produces an area of decreased density. In addition, the CT scan may help to define the location and size of the lesion (e.g., cortical versus subcortical infarctions), as well as small-vessel versus large-vessel disease.

1. The CT scan is positive in virtually all cases of intracerebral hemorrhage (increased density), and often shows interhemispheric blood or bleeding into brain parenchyma in subarachnoid hemorrhage. These changes are evident within the first hour after onset of symptoms. With CT scanning, patients with the clinical diagnosis of thrombosis often have intracerebral hemorrhage.

2. The CT scan is often negative for infarction in the first day after stroke, but focal low density may be evident 24 to 48 hours after the onset of symptoms. With contrast enhancement, infarction may mimic tumor on CT scan. However, the enhancement is generally not associated with the significant mass effect that occurs with enhancement of brain tumors.

3. Hemorrhagic infarction is often secondary to a large embolus. This produces increased density in CT scan. Anticoagulation should be delayed initially when hemorrhage is associated with embolic infarction.

4. Brainstem hemorrhage is usually visible on CT scan, but brainstem infarction may not be visible because of bony artifact at the base of the skull.

MAGNETIC RESONANCE IMAGING

MRI often reveals cerebral ischemia in its early stages, before it is visible on CT and often when the CT scan remains negative. MRI frequently will reveal brainstem, cerebellar, or temporal lobe infarctions not visible on CT scan. MRI is more accurate than CT in its ability to detect venous thrombosis as a cause of infarction. MRI is more sensitive in detecting small infarctions (e.g., lacunes). Diffusion-weighted MRI is the most sensitive technique in acute infarction. MRA may be used as a screen for extracranial arterial stenosis, but it may overestimate the degree of stenosis. It is accurate in predicting total vessel occlusion and is helpful in assessing the posterior circulation (vertebrobasilar) system. It is not accurate in assessing intracranial arterial stenosis. MRA and MRI in combination may show the location, size, and potentially the mechanism of stroke with one test. This combination of tests is most useful in thrombotic strokes, but may also be helpful in embolic strokes, lacunes, and hemorrhages. Because of the duration of the study, uncooperative patients may be difficult to image without sedation or anesthesia. In addition, patients who are unstable may not be good candidates for such scanning.

CT remains preferable to MRI in the acute stroke patient when hemorrhage is a consideration and when patient cooperation is a problem. In addition, MRI is often not the first choice for patients with acute stroke because (i) patients are acutely ill and not as easily monitored as with CT, (ii) CT is faster and more readily available, (iii) CT is better in the patient with claustrophobia, and (iv) CT is the benchmark study in assessing patients in acute stroke trials.

NONINVASIVE VASCULAR TESTING

1. High-resolution color-flow duplex ultrasonography (DU) is a low-cost, risk-free, noninvasive technology that can provide useful information about the degree of carotid stenosis. In good laboratories, DU has achieved accuracy, sensitivity, and specificity of more than 90% when compared to percutaneous cutfilm cerebral angiography. When the visualization is good, DU may also provide important information about plaque morphology (hemorrhage, cavitation, calcification, and stability), which may be important in determining the potential stroke risk. Because angiography is associated with a 1% to 2% risk of stroke or MI, many centers with validated laboratories have moved to using DU and MRA or CTa in concert to determine which patients may benefit from carotid endarterectomy.

2. TCD imaging allows assessment of the blood-flow characteristics of vessels in and about the circle of Willis. Because this region is not interrogated by DU, TCD is useful in assessing intracranial stenosis of the middle cerebral artery or vertebrobasilar system. TCD is technician dependent, and accuracy when compared to angiography may range from 60% to 85%. In addition, TCD is useful in assessing vasospasm in patients who have suffered subarachnoid hemorrhage from rupture of intracranial aneurysm. This largely has replaced angiography in the clinical setting because it is highly accurate (exceeding 90% sensitivity and specificity), is inexpensive, and can be done at the bedside at regular intervals to help guide the clinical management of these patients.

ARTERIOGRAPHY

Arteriography, by conventional or digital method, is performed (i) to identify surgically correctable lesions (e.g., intracranial aneurysms and AVMs, carotid artery stenosis, and ulcerated carotid plaques), (ii) to clarify an uncertain diagnosis, and (iii) sometimes when anticoagulation is planned to be more certain of the diagnosis. In guiding arteriography, it is important to decide clinically whether disease is in the carotid or vertebrobasilar system. Wherever possible, arteriography should be done by selective catheterization techniques by an experienced radiologist. The cost and small but definite risk of stroke and other adverse reactions during arteriography must be weighed against the clinical value of the test in each patient.

CTa provides information about extracranial and intracranial vessels that may reduce the need for formal angiography. Intravenous dye is used for this study, with its attendant risks. CTa may be obtained rapidly and can be used as part of rapid stroke assessment.

ECHOCARDIOGRAPHY

Echocardiography is useful in patients with a suspected cardiac-source embolization. Transthoracic echocardiography has limited sensitivity to identify sources of embolism but may be positive with ventricular mural thrombi, large vegetations, valvular lesions, and congenital heart disease. "Bubble studies" may show right-to-left shunts, which potentiate paradoxic embolization. Transesophageal echocardiography often shows sources of embolism not visualized with transthoracic echo and is most helpful in young patients without obvious risk factors for stroke.

LUMBAR PUNCTURE

With the advent of CT scan, lumbar punctures are performed infrequently in the evaluation of the stroke patient. A lumbar puncture (see Chapter 30) is performed in the following situations:

- Meningitis is suspected.
- Subarachnoid hemorrhage is a diagnostic possibility. CT scans may be falsely negative in 5% to 10% of patients with subarachnoid hemorrhage. Subarachnoid hemorrhage shows grossly bloody CSF and usually an elevated CSF pressure.

TREATMENT

Risk factor modification and cholesterol-lowering regimens are key components of stroke treatment. Appropriate attention to smoking cessation, blood pressure, and diabetes control are crucial. HMG-CoA (3-hydroxy-3-methylglutaryl coenzyme A) reductase agents may reduce the risk of recurrent stroke by 30%, with or without hypercholesterolemia. There also has been recognition of the value of weight reduction, aerobic exercise, and proper diet in stroke prevention.

CARDIAC EMBOLI: ANTICOAGULATION

Anticoagulation is beneficial in preventing further embolization in patients with cardiac emboli (unless the source is bacterial endocarditis). Thus diagnosing an embolus of cardiac origin is crucial. It is important to perform a CT scan or MRI to rule out bleeding before beginning anticoagulation. The timing of anticoagulation after embolism remains controversial. Immediate anticoagulation therapy in patients with acute ischemic stroke is not associated with any short-term benefit. Recurrent embolus in the days after cardiac embolism occurs at a low rate, and the benefit of immediate anticoagulation seems to be counterbalanced by the risk of major bleeding. Particular caution and delay in anticoagulation are advised in elderly patients and in those with massive infarcts (greater than 5 cm in diameter) and uncontrolled hypertension. Begin with heparin, then switch to warfarin. An international normalization ratio (INR) of 2.0 to 3.0 appears to be required for effective stroke prevention in these patients. Higher levels of anticoagulation may be necessary for patients with metal prosthetic valves. If the embolus is caused by a mural thrombus associated with an MI, anticoagulation is usually continued for 6 months. If atrial fibrillation or rheumatic valvular disease is the cause, long-term anticoagulation is indicated.

CAROTID STENOSIS

1. *Asymptomatic extracranial carotid stenosis:* In patients with severe asymptomatic carotid stenosis, the risk of stroke is 2% per year with medical management alone. Less than 60% diameter stenosis is treated medically. In patients with more than 60% diameter stenosis, a large multicenter study (Asymptomatic Carotid Atherosclerosis Study, or ACAS) showed reduction of stroke from 2% to 1% per year in good-risk patients who underwent surgery. This favorable result depended on a surgical and angiographic morbidity and mortality of less than 3%.

2. *Symptomatic extracranial carotid stenosis:* The risk of stroke increases with increasing degrees of carotid stenosis. A large

multicenter study (North American Symptomatic Carotid Endarterectomy Trial, or NASCET) showed benefit of carotid surgery in medically stable patients with angiographically demonstrated 70% or greater diameter stenosis. Certain sub-groups of symptomatic patients with moderate carotid stenosis (50% to 70%) benefit from surgery provided there is low sur-gical morbidity and mortality. Carotid stenting is now available at many centers. However, published results from stenting series still do not reach the low level of risk of carotid endarterectomy in medically stable patients, though the risks of this procedure are trending down. Patients who require a carotid procedure but who cannot undergo surgery may be stenting candidates.

3. *Completed carotid occlusion and stroke:* With completed carotid occlusion and stroke, urgent surgery appears to be of little benefit and may convert a bland infarction into a hemorrhagic one unless the surgery is performed within minutes of the stroke. Extracranial–intracranial vascular bypass has been found to be of no benefit in a large multicenter study. Similarly, short-term anticoagulation is used in many patients, but its value has not been proved in randomized studies.

SMALL-VESSEL LACUNAR STROKES

Antiplatelet therapy including aspirin, clopidogrel, or ASA/dipyridamole is usually used to treat small-vessel lacunar strokes (see Chapter 16). In addition, risk factor modification is probably critical. There have been no major trials of therapy in patients with only small-vessel ischemic stroke.

GENERAL CARE OF COMPLETED INFARCTION

1. Treatment in a specialized "stroke unit" is cost effective and improves outcome from stroke.
2. Urgent assessment of clinical status is imperative in throm-botic stroke. Newer agents are available that, in some cases, may change the course of the completed infarction.
3. In selected cases, tissue plasminogen activator (tPA) given intravenously according to a specific protocol appears to improve the functional outcome at 3 months in patients with moderate-sized infarctions of various mechanisms. In a multi-center trial, tPA appeared to be effective only when given in

the first 3 hours after stroke. The hemorrhage rate in treated patients was 6.3% compared with placebo, in which the rate was less than 1%. tPA should be administered only under the supervision of physicians experienced in its use in stroke and only when neurosurgical consultation is available.

4. Aspirin has been studied extensively for secondary prevention of stroke and reduces risk of nonfatal stroke, MI, and death by approximately 25% in most studies in patients with prior stroke or TIA. Clopidogrel (75 mg/day) and ASA/dipyridamole have slightly greater efficacy than aspirin in secondary stroke prevention.

5. Careful monitoring of the patient's status, attention to details of nursing such as prevention of deep vein thrombosis and decubiti, and prevention of aspiration from dysphagia are important in completed stroke.

6. Excessive blood pressure elevation should be treated cautiously. Moderate blood pressure elevation should not be treated because this may be a beneficial response to at-risk ischemic areas and often resolves on its own. Aggressive blood pressure treatment in the setting of acute infarction may cause a worsening of the stroke deficit because of further ischemia. Further studies are needed to assess the role of acute blood pressure management after ischemic stroke.

7. In patients with herniation, treatment with agents that reduce intracranial pressure may be helpful. Cranioplasty and duraplasty may be used as a rescue treatment for patients with major strokes who have massive life-threatening edema.

8. Cerebellar infarction with mass effect is a neurosurgical emergency. Immediate decompression may be life saving.

9. Heparinization should be avoided in large infarctions because of the risk of hemorrhage.

   Despite having been used in stroke therapy for years, heparin remains of unproven efficacy in the prevention of stroke or recurrent infarction.

SUBARACHNOID HEMORRHAGE, SUBDURAL AND EPIDURAL HEMORRHAGE

Treatment of subarachnoid hemorrhage caused by aneurysm includes strict bed rest; control of blood pressure; and careful medical management including electrolyte monitoring, stool softeners, analgesia, and, whenever possible, early surgical clipping of the aneurysm. Without appropriate treatment, approximately

50% of those patients with subarachnoid hemorrhage who survive the first 24 hours will die within the next 2 weeks. The clinical condition of the patient, the presence of arterial spasm, and the location of the aneurysm influence surgical intervention. Vasospasm (narrowing of blood vessels on arteriography plus neurologic symptoms) usually begins 3 to 14 days after the initial bleed. Nimodipine, a calcium antagonist, reduces cerebral arterial vasospasm and is usually started immediately. There is a definite trend toward "early" aneurysm surgery after subarachnoid hemorrhage followed by volume expansion and elevation of blood pressure in an attempt to prevent rebleeding and to reduce vasospasm. Endovascular placement of coils in aneurysms has been shown to be superior to surgery in selected cases with small, accessible aneurysms.

INTRACEREBRAL HEMORRHAGE

Treatment of increased intracranial pressure, stabilization of blood pressure, and consideration of neurosurgical decompression are important. Steroids have not been shown to be useful in the treatment of intracerebral hemorrhage. Non-dominant putaminal hemorrhages or lobar hemorrhages with a risk of herniation may be helped by evacuation of the clot. Cerebellar hemorrhages with brainstem compression should be decompressed rapidly, if possible, to prevent irreversible brainstem injury. Massive intracerebral hemorrhages with brain injury are unlikely to be helped even with aggressive surgical treatment. Remember, identification of the cause of the hemorrhage and its mechanism (e.g., coagulopathy) is critical. Recent trials using recombinant factor VII in patients with acute intracerebral hemorrhage before 6 hours have shown a decrease in mortality but at the risk of increased thrombotic events due to increased clotting.

RECOVERY

Rehabilitation begins in the hospital as soon as possible and is best delivered as a comprehensive group of services tailored to the individual patient's needs. There is extensive literature supporting inpatient and outpatient rehabilitation in stroke patients. Functional recovery is improved by the early recognition and treatment of depression, which is common in stroke.

Suggested Readings

Adams HP, Adams RJ, Brott T, et al. Guidelines for the early management of patients with ischemic stroke. *Stroke*. 2003;34: 1056–1083.

Aguilar MI, Hart RG, Kase CS, et al. Treatment of warfarin-associated intracerebral hemorrhage: literature review and expert opinion. *Mayo Clin Proc*. 2007;82:387.

Albers GW, Amarenco P, Easton JD, et al. Antithrombotic and thrombolytic therapy for ischemic stroke: the seventh ACCP conference on antithrombotic and thrombolytic therapy. *Chest*. 2004;126:483S–512S.

deOliveira JG, Beck J, Ulrich C, et al. Comparison between clipping and coiling on the incidence of cerebral vasospasm after aneurismal subarachnoid hemorrhage: a systematic review and meta-analysis. *Neurosurg Rev*. 2007;30:22–30.

Gubitz G, Counsell C, Sandercock P, et al. Anticoagulants for acute ischaemic stoke (Cochrane Review). In: Cochrane Library Issue 1, 2003. Oxford: Update Software.

Mohr JP, Thomas JC, Lazar RM, et al. A comparison of warfarin and aspirin for prevention of recurrent ischemic stroke. *N Engl J Med*. 2001;345:1444–1451.

Molyneux A, Kerr R, Stratton I, et al. International subarachnoid aneurysm trial of neurosurgical clipping versus endovascular coils in 2143 patients with ruptured intracerebral aneurysms: a randomized trial. *Lancet*. 2002;360:267–274.

16 Selected Stroke Syndromes

CASE

A 67-year-old hypertensive male smoker comes in with sudden onset of complete paralysis of the right side of the body. His right face is weak, and his speech is slurred. Despite this, he is completely aware of his surroundings and has normal memory and affect. His sensory exam is normal. His right toe is upgoing.

Diagnosis

Lacunar infarction, left internal capsule, with pure motor hemiparesis.

LACUNAR INFARCTION

Lacunes are vascular lesions in the brain commonly seen in patients with hypertension or diabetes. They are small areas of thrombotic infarction that become pea-sized holes pathologically. It is important to recognize lacunar strokes, because they represent small-vessel disease and generally require limited investigation. Control of hypertension, hyperglycemia, hyperlipidemia, cessation of smoking, and use of antiplatelet agents are likely to improve outcome and prevent future strokes.

Look for these characteristic syndromes:

1. *Pure motor hemiplegia*, in which there is a lesion in the pons or internal capsule. Paralysis of face, arm, and leg without sensory loss. A right hemiplegia of lacunar origin that has no accompanying aphasia. With a left hemiplegia, there are no parietal lobe findings.
2. *Pure sensory stroke*, in which there is a lesion most often in the thalamus. Contralateral sensory loss in the face, arm, and leg, with no hemiplegia or other signs. **Thalamic sensory loss may cause a loss of pin sensation affecting one side that splits the midline.**
3. *Clumsy-hand dysarthria*, showing a lesion in the pons or internal capsule. Slurred speech with clumsiness and mild weakness of one arm.

4. *Crural (leg) paresis and ataxia (ataxic hemiparesis)* with a lesion in the pons, or internal capsule. Ataxia and weakness of one leg.

INTRACEREBRAL HEMORRHAGE

Computed tomography (CT) scan is diagnostic in acute intracerebral hemorrhage.

Note: CT may miss hemorrhage in the brainstem and cerebellum because of bony artifacts. If the CT is "normal" and a clinical suspicion of posterior circulation hemorrhage remains, a magnetic resonance imaging scan should be obtained.

Cerebellar Hemorrhage

Cerebellar hemorrhage is important to diagnose because it can lead to rapid death via brainstem compression; treatment is surgical evacuation of the clot. Headache, vomiting, and inability to walk with normal lower-extremity strength are cardinal features. Strength and sensation are usually normal (unless brainstem compression occurs). The patient may have trouble looking to the side of the lesion (gaze paresis). Nystagmus and limb ataxia may not be present. Ipsilateral facial weakness may be present. Cerebellar infarction with subsequent swelling may mimic cerebellar hemorrhage, and require surgical treatment.

Putaminal

Most intracerebral hemorrhages occur in the *putamen*. Look for the following:

1. Hemiplegia.
2. Striking eye deviation to side of hemorrhage and away from the hemiplegia (Fig. 16.1).
3. Headache.
4. Homonymous visual field deficit contralateral to the lesion.
5. Cortical deficits, which develop as the hemorrhage progresses.

Thalamic

May or may not have hemiplegia. Has eyes that look down at the nose, with small and nonreactive pupils (Fig. 16.1). Has marked contralateral sensory loss.

Right putaminal hemorrhage

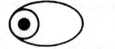

Eyes deviate to the side of the lesion.
Pupils: normal size and reactive.
(seen also with large hemisphere infarcts)

Thalamic hemorrhage

Eyes look down at the nose; vertical gaze is
impaired. Pupils: small and nonreactive.

Pontine hemorrhage

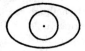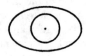

Eyes are midposition with no movement to doll's
eyes maneuver. There may be ocular bobbing.
Pupils: pinpoint, react to light if viewed with a
magnifying glass.

Cerebellar hemorrhage

Patient has difficulty looking to the side of the
lesion. There may be skew deviation or a sixth
nerve palsy. Pupils: normal size and reactive.

FIGURE 16.1. Eye signs in intracerebral hemorrhage.

PONTINE HEMORRHAGE

The patient is comatose with small pinpoint pupils (Fig. 16.1).
Pupils react to bright light when viewed with a magnifying glass.
There is quadriparesis, with upgoing toes. Patient has no horizontal

extraocular movements with passive head turning or use of ice-water calorics. Ocular bobbing may occur (rapid downward eye deflection with slow upward drift). The patient may be locked-in (conscious, but unable to move to show consciousness). He or she may retain the ability to look up and down.

Note: The most common causes of intracerebral hemorrhage are hypertension and trauma. Other causes include blood dyscrasias, side effects of anticoagulant therapy, drug abuse (cocaine), amyloid angiopathy, brain tumors, and cryptic arterio-venous malformations (AVMs).

SUBARACHNOID HEMORRHAGE

Subarachnoid hemorrhage (SAH) classically presents with the sudden onset of severe headache during activity, altered level of consciousness; at times, coma, nuchal rigidity, and bloody cere-brospinal fluid. There may be autonomic disturbances such as vomiting, fever, and electrocardiogram changes. Hemorrhage into the brain substance appears as an increased density on CT scan; arterial spasm generally produces no changes on CT scan. Delayed deterioration in patients with SAH may be caused by hydro-cephalus, seizures, cerebral edema, vasospasm, or rebleeding.

The most common locations for aneurysms are at various arterial junction points around the circle of Willis at the base of the brain:

1. Posterior communicating artery: may have associated third nerve palsy.
2. Anterior communicating artery: mutism and leg weakness may occur.
3. Middle cerebral artery: aphasia or nondominant hemisphere findings.
4. Less common locations include ophthalmic artery (unilateral blindness), cavernous sinus (ophthalmoplegia), and basilar artery (brainstem signs).

Note: **CT scan is abnormal in 90% of cases of SAH, and has a false-negative rate of 10%. Therefore, do a lumbar puncture in suspected SAH when CT is "normal."**

BRAIN ARTERIOVENOUS MALFORMATIONS

These are the most dangerous congenital malformations. They occur in about 0.1% of the population, and 90% are in the supra-tentorial compartment.

These malformations cause symptoms by causing:

1. Intracerebral hemorrhage or subarachnoid hemorrhage.
2. Seizures.
3. Focal neurologic deficits.
4. Headaches.

The size can range from a few millimeters to an entire hemisphere. MRI or CT can make the diagnosis, but angiography is needed to precisely define the vascular territories supplying the AVM in planning therapy.

Treatment is complex, because the natural history of AVMs varies, and the treatments available run the risk of causing neurologic deficits in some patients. Treatments include:

1. Stereotactic radiosurgery.
2. Endovascular embolization.
3. Surgery.

Treatment of seizures is similar to that of other patients with epilepsy.

FOCAL THROMBOEMBOLIC STROKES

The *middle cerebral artery syndrome* seldom is caused by thrombosis of the middle cerebral artery; it is usually secondary to an occluded carotid in the neck or an embolus to the middle cerebral artery. Look for the following:

- Hemiparesis (greater in face and arm than in leg).
- Aphasia or nondominant hemisphere findings (depending on the side).
- Cortical sensory loss (greater in face and arm than in leg).
- Homonymous hemianopsia.
- Conjugate eye deviation (to the side of the hemisphere lesion).

"Partial" middle cerebral artery syndromes, almost always of embolic origin, may include:

1. Sensorimotor paresis with little aphasia.
2. Conduction aphasia.
3. Wernicke aphasia without hemiparesis.

In the anterior cerebral artery syndrome, look for the following:

- Paralysis of the lower extremity.
- Cortical sensory loss in leg only.

- Incontinence.
- Grasp and suck reflexes.
- Slowness in mentation with perseveration.
- No hemianopsia or aphasia.
- Limb apraxia.

Occlusion of the *internal carotid artery* gives a picture resembling occlusion of the middle cerebral artery. When the anterior cerebral territory is included in the area of infarction, clinical features of anterior cerebral occlusion also occur.

Posterior cerebral artery syndrome presents these features:

- Homonymous hemianopsia (often the only finding); the patient may be unaware of the deficit.
- Little or no paralysis.
- Occasional prominent sensory loss, including to pinprick and touch, due to thalamic perforator involvement.
- No aphasia or nondominant hemisphere dysfunction.

Also, patients with left posterior cerebral artery syndrome may be unable to read, but still may be able to write (alexia without agraphia). Recent memory loss may be present (involvement of hippocampus). Occasionally, patients with posterior cerebral artery syndromes can have a loss of color vision, difficulty recognizing faces (prosopagnosia), and with bilateral occipital infarction, may be blind, but unaware of this deficit (Anton syndrome).

Watershed or *border zone infarction syndromes* (common after anoxia) include proximal arm weakness with distal sparing and transcortical aphasia (see Chapter 4).

Brainstem syndromes never have cortical deficits or visual field defects. One of the most common brainstem syndromes is the *lateral medullary (Wallenberg syndrome)*, caused by occlusion of the vertebral or posterior inferior cerebellar artery (see Fig. 34.9). Look for the following:

- Ipsilateral to the lesion: facial numbness, limb ataxia, Horner syndrome (miosis, ptosis, anhidrosis), pain over the eye (spinal tract of V, cerebellar peduncle, sympathetic pathways).
- Contralateral to the lesion: pinprick and temperature loss in arm and leg (spinothalamic tract).
- Vertigo, nausea, hiccups, hoarseness, difficulty swallowing (ninth and tenth nerve nuclei).
- If the lesion is typical, treatment is supportive, and these patients usually do well.

Beware of aspiration in Wallenberg syndrome because of swallowing difficulty.

TABLE 16.1. Named Brainstem Syndromes

Eponym	Site	Cranial Nerves	Tracts	Signs	Usual Cause
Weber	Base of midbrain	III	Corticospinal	Oculomotor palsy with crossed hemiplegia	Vascular, tumor
Claude	Midbrain tegmentum	III	Red nucleus and brachium conjunctivum	Oculomotor palsy with contralateral cerebellar ataxia and tremor	Vascular, tumor
Benedict	Midbrain tegmentum	III	Red nucleus, corticospinal tract, brachium conjunctivum	Oculomotor palsy, contralateral cerebellar ataxia, corticospinal signs	Vascular, tuberculoma, tumor
Nothnagel	Midbrain tectum	Unilateral or bilateral III	Superior cerebellar peduncles	Ocular palsies, paralysis of gaze, cerebellar ataxia	Tumor
Parinaud	Dorsal midbrain			Paralysis of upward gaze and accommodation, fixed pupil, retraction nystagmus	Pinealoma, hydrocephalus
Millard–Gubler and Raymond–Foville	Base of pons	VII and sometimes VI	Corticospinal tract	Facial and 6th-nerve palsy, contralateral hemiplegia, sometimes gaze palsy	Vascular, tumor
Avellis	Medulla tegmentum	X	Spinothalamic, sometimes pupillary fibers	Paralysis of soft palate and vocal cord and contralateral hemianesthesia	Infarct or tumor
Jackson	Medulla tegmentum	X, XII	Corticospinal	Avellis plus ipsilateral tongue	Infarct or tumor
Wallenberg	Medulla, lateral tegmentum	Spinal V, IV, X, XI	Lateral STT, descending pupil fibers, spinocerebellar and olivocerebellar tracts	Ipsi V, IV, X, XI palsy, Horner, cerebellar ataxia. Contra pain and temp	Vascular—pica or vertebral

Table reproduced with permission from Dr. Timothy Hain. Source: www.dizziness-and-balance.com/disorders/central/brainstem%20strokes.htm.

There are a variety of other named brainstem syndromes defined by their distribution and the cranial nerves involved (see Table 16.1).

Most other brainstem strokes are in the *pons* (see Fig. 34.8).

1. If the lesion is in the *medial* portion of the pons, there is weakness and an internuclear ophthalmoplegia or gaze palsy with little sensory loss.
2. If the lesion is in the *lateral and tegmental* portion of the pons, sensory loss predominates.
3. *Cerebellar* signs are present in lateral lesions, and are ipsilateral to the lesion.
4. Midbrain strokes frequently involve the third nerve, or nucleus and cerebral peduncle, thus producing ipsilateral pupil dilatation, ptosis, ophthalmoparesis, and contralateral hemiplegia (Weber syndrome; see Fig. 34.7). Occasionally, retraction-convergence nystagmus (when the patient looks up, the eyes converge and retract intermittently) occurs.

Suggested Readings

Freeman WD, Brott TG. Modern treatment options for intracerebral hemorrhage. *Curr Treat Options Neurol.* 2006;8:145–157.

Mendelow AD, Unterberg A. Surgical treatment of intracerebral haemorrhage. *Curr Opin Crit Care.* 2007;1:169–174.

Sacco S, Marini C, Totaro R. A population-based study of the incidence and prognosis of lacunar stroke. *Neurology.* 2006;66:1335–1338.

17 Transient Ischemic Attack

CASE

A 62-year-old, right-handed pipe fitter, with hypertension, hyperlipidemia, and coronary artery disease, develops a sudden onset of right-sided weakness of the arm and leg, a facial droop on the right side, and difficulty "getting his words out." These symptoms last for 15 minutes and resolve completely. In the ED, his exam is normal except for bilateral femoral bruits and a blood pressure of 160/90. Carotid ultrasound shows preocclusive stenosis of both carotid arteries at the bifurcations.

Diagnosis

TIA, left hemisphere, due to preocclusive carotid stenosis.

Transient ischemic attack (TIA) is an acute neurologic deficit of vascular origin that clears completely. It usually lasts anywhere from several minutes to an hour, but by current definition remains no more than 24 hours. Recent data indicate that deficits lasting more than 60 minutes, even if symptoms resolve, represent infarctions when studied with MRI. TIAs are a symptom of disease, not a specific disorder. Half to two-thirds of people with thrombotic strokes give a history of a previous TIA, and approximately one-fourth of patients with TIAs will have a stroke within 3 years. Many of these strokes occur within 2 days of the TIA.

The following points should be established in the patient with a TIA.

IS THE TIA DUE TO ARTERIAL DISEASE IN THE CAROTID OR VERTEBROBASILAR TERRITORY?

1. *TIAs in carotid distribution*. Transient monocular blindness in the eye on the same side as a stenosed internal carotid artery (amaurosis fugax). The patient may report a "shade coming down" over the eye or obscuration that appears like "white steam" over one eye.

- Transient aphasia.
- Motor and sensory symptoms in a single extremity (upper or lower), involving face and arm (middle cerebral artery–territory involvement), or a clumsy ("bear paw") hand.

2. *TIAs in vertebrobasilar distribution.* Slurred speech, dizziness, diplopia, ataxia, syncope, loss of consciousness, dysphagia, numbness around lips or face.
   - Hemiparesis and hemisensory loss do not parallel each other in the individual limb as in carotid disease.
   - There may be bilateral motor or sensory deficits from a single lesion.

3. *Lacunar or small-vessel thrombotic strokes.* Occur abruptly, or in a stuttering fashion over hours or days. There may be a warning. Headache is absent, and risk factors such as hypertension, smoking, hyperlipidemia, and diabetes are usually present.

TIAs in *carotid territory* usually are associated with severe stenosis, but may be associated with moderate stenosis and ulcerative plaque at the carotid bifurcation in the neck. With carotid symptoms, especially in association with a carotid bruit or decreased carotid pulse, noninvasive carotid evaluation using carotid duplex ultrasound, CT angiography, or magnetic resonance angiography (MRA) are performed to define the vascular anatomy, and to determine whether the patient is a candidate for carotid endarterectomy. Recently stenting of the carotids has emerged, but is still reserved for medically unstable patients with symptomatic disease. Occasionally, traditional cerebral arteriography may be necessary if the vascular anatomy is not well imaged with non-invasive techniques. Remember, the carotid must have a 75% cross-sectional area reduction before the blood flow is decreased significantly. If the TIA is caused by emboli from an ulcerated plaque, stenosis need not be present. There are patients who have an occluded internal carotid with no symptoms at all. Moreover, patients may have a carotid bruit without stenosis and stenosis without a bruit.

TIAs in the *vertebrobasilar territory, the vertebral arteries, and their origins* have a predilection for atheroma development. Emboli of cardiac origin to the vertebrobasilar territory occur, as does artery-to-artery embolism. Serious vertebrobasilar disease may be intracranial, in which surgery is not feasible, and the benefit of operation on the vertebral arteries in the neck is unproven. Stenting can be performed with intracranial and extracranial vertebrobasilar disease, but the risks of this procedure are significant, and must be weighed against medical treatment.

Vertigo alone is rarely a symptom of vertebrobasilar insufficiency, unless other brainstem signs or symptoms are present. Occasionally, an elderly patient may have vertebrobasilar symptoms when turning the head, these being secondary to mechanical factors in the cervical region that reduce blood flow.

IS THE HEART THE SOURCE OF THE TIA?

Emboli from the heart are well-recognized causes of TIAs, and are seen with a variety of cardiac sources of emboli. Cardiac emboli may cause TIAs, but they may be in different territories (e.g., first an episode of right-sided weakness, then an episode of left-sided weakness). Transesophageal echocardiography (TEE) is particularly helpful for detecting cardiac embolic sources, such as mural thrombi or emboli from atherosclerosis in the ascending aorta. In addition, anomalies of the atria such as atrial septal aneurysm and atrial septal defect are imaged using TEE.

Patients with atrial fibrillation may have TIA.

DIFFERENTIAL DIAGNOSIS OF TRANSIENT NEUROLOGIC DYSFUNCTION

There are a handful of other pathophysiologic processes that cause transient neurologic dysfunction lasting minutes. These can be mistaken for TIA, but have a completely different implication for treatment and workup. Anytime there are transient neurologic symptoms these should be considered.

1. *Seizure* (see Chapter 20). Keep in mind that focal seizures may produce transient neurologic symptoms (numbness, leg or arm movement, or weakness). The deficit is usually brief, lasting seconds unless there is focal status epilepticus. Obtain an electroencephalogram (EEG) if seizures are suspected.
2. *Migraine* (see Chapter 18). Of special note, migraine may be accompanied by transient neurologic signs or symptoms (visual disturbances, motor or sensory). They usually can be identified by the headache that follows the neurologic deficit, and by the gastrointestinal symptoms. It appears in patients younger than those with cerebrovascular disease. Nevertheless, older people experience migrainous phenomena, and there may be no accompanying headache (e.g., "typical aura without headache"). Thus, migraine variants in the elderly post a difficult diagnostic

and therapeutic problem. Migrainous sensory symptoms often "march" along an extremity. The time course of migraine aura is usually minutes, and there are usually some "positive symptoms" such as flashing lights, tingling, and the like. Patients can experience episodic vertigo, and occasionally lateralized neurologic symptoms, such as altered speech or weakness on one side.

3. *Transient global amnesia* (TGA). A unique syndrome in which, typically, a middle-aged patient suddenly loses recent memory, becomes confused, and asks the same questions repeatedly. The patient appears alert; has no motor or sensory signs or symptoms; and retains "personal identity" and the ability to answer questions about job, address, and so on. A characteristic feature is the repetition of the same questions by the patient despite being given the answer. The etiology of this dramatic syndrome is unknown, but it is not a risk factor for stroke. TGA is associated with hypertension or a history of migraine. Attacks of TGA are often triggered by special circumstances, such as emotional experiences, pain, or sexual intercourse. Attacks usually last hours and clear without residual deficit. Unless attacks are recurrent, which is rare, treatment is unnecessary.

4. In patients with MS, there may be *transient neurologic episodes* (TNE). These episodes consist of lasting seconds of focal numbness, weakness, twitching, vertigo, diplopia, or dysarthria. These may occur hundreds of times a day, and last only seconds. They are due to axonal cross-talk (ephaptic transmission) due to demyelination. Such spells may be the first manifestation of MS.

5. *Hypoglycemia*. Patients with hypoglycemia may have neurologic symptoms, but the setting and attendant autonomic symptoms in a diabetic are usually diagnostic.

6. *Hyperventilation*. This may cause neurologic symptoms of tingling, often in a peripheral and perioral distribution. Having the patient hyperventilate is very useful in recreating the symptoms. However, hyperventilation will also bring out symptoms in patients with MS having TNE.

7. *Syncope:* See Chapter 20.

TREATMENT OF THE PATIENT WITH TIA

1. After a complete workup, including:

   - Electrocardiogram.
   - Holter monitor or echocardiography.
   - Auscultation for bruits.

- Blood pressure check in both arms.
- Noninvasive tests such as duplex ultrasound, MRA, and rarely, EEG.

Arteriography may be necessary before deciding on a mode of treatment. Frequently, a combination of noninvasive vascular testing and MRA, or cerebral tomographic angiography, is replacing angiography in preoperative assessment for carotid endarterectomy. It is *critical* for the clinician to determine the cause of the transient neurologic deficit (e.g., embolism, migraine, arrhythmia) before embarking on a course of therapy.

2. Carotid endarterectomy is indicated when there is a unilateral severely stenosed (70%–99% diameter stenosis) carotid in a patient with TIAs in that vessel's territory. However, only if the surgery can be done with less than a 3% morbidity and mortality rate.
3. Anticoagulation is indicated for patients with cardioembolic TIAs, or where there is a coagulopathy causing TIA. Heparin often is used in patients with preocclusive stenosis after a TIA while awaiting surgery. However, there are no convincing data to support this practice.
4. For those who have an ulcerated or irregular plaque, without severe stenosis that may form the nidus of embolic material, or in those with small-vessel disease, antiplatelet agents are used (e.g., aspirin, ASA/dipyridamole, or clopidogrel).
5. There is no evidence that anticoagulation benefits patients with small-vessel disease, a completed stroke, or a completely occluded large vessel. Despite this, patients with acute carotid occlusion are frequently placed on coumadin for a few months to reduce the risk of embolic from the carotid "stump."
6. Data from the warfarin versus aspirin in recurrent stroke study (WARSS) did not indicate a benefit of coumadin over aspirin for patients with large-vessel stenotic lesions (see Mohr et al., 2001).

Suggested Readings

Algra A, de Schryver EL, van Gijn J, et al. Oral anticoagulants versus antiplatelet therapy for preventing further vascular events after transient ischaemic attack or minor stroke of presumed arterial origin. *Cochrane Database Syst Rev.* 2006;3: CD001342.
Hodges JR. Unraveling the enigma of transient global amnesia. *Ann Neurol.* 1998;43:151–153.

Lamonte MP. Evaluation and management of transient ischemic attacks. *Clin Geriatr Med*. 2007;23:401–412.

Mohr JP, Thomas JC, Lazar RM, et al. A comparison of warfarin and aspirin for prevention of recurrent ischemic stroke. *N Engl J Med*. 2001;345:1444–1451.

Sylaja PN, Hill MD. Current management of transient ischemic attack. *Am J Cardiovasc Drugs*. 2007;7:67–74.

18 Headache

CASE

A 24-year-old law student comes to your office with headache. Once or twice a month, she develops a severe, left-sided, hemicranial pounding headache that lasts for a few hours. When she goes to sleep, it is gone by the time she wakes up. On rare occasions, she sees spots and zig-zag lines during her headache. She responds well to an oral triptan and an anti-inflammatory medication.

Diagnosis

Migraine with and without visual aura.

Headache is common, often banal, but sometimes caused by life-threatening disease. Taking a history that reviews the features of the headache syndrome is the key to diagnosis. It is important to distinguish the three major types of "benign" headache (migraine, cluster, and tension-type headache), and to recognize the warning symptoms and signs of more ominous headaches. Features that provide crucial information include the character of the headache, its timing and duration, exacerbating and relieving factors, and associated symptoms.

THE CHARACTER OF THE HEADACHE

Migraine headaches are periodic, throbbing headaches; usually unilateral, and over one eye or in the temple. Sensitivity to sound (phonophobia) and light (photophobia) is common, as are nausea and vomiting. Scalp sensitivity is also common. Neurologic symptoms may precede the headache (migraine with aura), or the headache may occur alone (migraine without aura). There is often a family history of migraine. Sometimes that patient has a history of motion sickness. Symptoms often begin during teenage years. Migraine is more common in females.

Cluster headaches are sharp, knife-like, and unilateral, and often are over one eye. They are more common in males, and begin later in life than do migraine headaches.

Tension-type headaches tend to be diffuse, steady, non-throbbing headaches in the front or back of the head. They are bilateral, and often described as "band-like," "pressure," or "tight" headaches. They occur in all age groups.

TIMING AND DURATION

Migraine headaches are periodic, lasting a few hours to a few days. They may occur at any time and may awaken the patient from sleep. They often begin during a "relaxed" time (e.g., the week-end). **Status migrainosus** refers to migraine that lasts for days.

Cluster headaches come in groups over a few weeks or months (a cluster), and then subside. They last for a few minutes to 1 to 2 hours and tend to occur at the same time every day. They may awaken the patient 1 or 2 hours after falling asleep.

Tension-type headaches usually last hours, but may last days, weeks, and even months. They frequently occur at the end of a stressful day.

EXACERBATING AND RELIEVING FACTORS

Migraine may be exacerbated or relieved during menstruation or pregnancy or at the time of menopause. Migraine is often relieved by sleep, or after vomiting. Migraine may be brought on by hunger, alcohol ingestion, caffeine withdrawal, and certain foods such as aged cheese, cured meats, and chocolate. The use of birth control pills may worsen migraine.

Cluster headaches are often precipitated by alcohol, sometimes exquisitely so. Cluster headaches are not relieved by environmental factors until they have run their course.

Tension-type headaches may be relieved with relaxation, neck massage, or rest.

ASSOCIATED SYMPTOMS

Migraine with aura may be accompanied by a variety of neuro-logic symptoms, often immediately preceding the headache. These include visual symptoms such as flashing lights, zig-zag lines, blind spots, or complete loss of a visual field. These last for minutes, and the headache usually begins as the visual symptoms recede. Many other neurologic symptoms can occur. These include visual field loss, difficulty talking, tingling of parts of the body, and even hemiparesis ("hemiplegic migraine"). Confusion, vertigo, stupor, and ataxia are less common but well-documented manifestations of migraine. A key feature that distinguishes migranous neurologic symptoms from stroke is their progression over minutes rather than seconds.

In *cluster* headaches, tearing, facial flushing, and a stuffy, runny nose are common. These are usually ipsilateral to the headache. Sometimes Horner syndrome may accompany the headache (small pupil, ptosis). These are all features of autonomic dysfunction.

Tension-type headaches lack associated symptoms.

OMINOUS HEADACHES

Occasionally, a patient presenting with a new or changed headache is harboring a major illness that requires diagnosis and treatment. The following symptoms are suggestive of an ominous cause and, if present, require careful evaluation:

1. A change in character, pattern, or timing of a preexisting headache.
2. A new-onset headache, especially after age 50.
3. Headache associated with persistent neurologic signs or symptoms.
4. A sudden, severe "worst headache of my life" (suggests SAH).
5. A progressive headache over days or weeks (mass lesion).
6. Stiff neck, fever, altered mental status (meningitis or encephalitis).
7. Headache with jaw pain, systemic symptoms, visual blurring (temporal arteritis).

EXAMINATION OF THE PATIENT WITH HEADACHE

Examination sometimes offers clues to the type of headache or to the presence of organic causes, especially if the patient is symptomatic during the examination.

In headache, the examination is usually negative.

1. Look carefully for *focal signs* suggesting a tumor or other structural lesions. (Make sure to check the fundi for papilledema).

2. Check for *autonomic dysfunction* during headache, for cluster (e.g., miotic pupil, ptosis, red eye, tearing, unilateral nasal congestion).
3. Check for *meningismus* (subarachnoid hemorrhage, meningitis).
4. Listen for *bruit* over one eye, skull, and neck (arteriovenous malformation, carotid-cavernous fistula, severe carotid stenosis).
5. Headache over the eye in a person older than 50 may be caused by *temporal arteritis*. Check for a tender temporal artery, or nodularity of the artery.
6. Note hypertension, which may exacerbate migraine or tension headaches, particularly if the hypertension is labile.
7. Glaucoma is a cause of headache in the elderly; headache, eye pain, red eye, and vomiting are common. Palpate the globe, and perform tonometry if glaucoma is suspected. Treatment with medication or eye surgery may prevent blindness. Thus, early diagnosis is crucial.
8. Constant headache in an obese female may be caused by pseudotumor cerebri. This is associated with papilledema as a result of increased intracranial pressure (see Chapter 30).
9. Occipital headache may be caused by cervical arthritis, especially in the elderly. Exacerbation of pain by neck movement is helpful in the diagnosis.
10. Headache precipitated by coughing or Valsalva may be due to a posterior fossa mass or a Chiari malformation.

Note: **Temporal arteritis and glaucoma may present as headache in the elderly, and either may lead to blindness.**

LABORATORY STUDIES

Laboratory studies in the patient with headache depend on the clinical impression after obtaining the history, and performing a careful examination. All headache sufferers probably should receive a complete blood count, chemistry screen, and sedimentation rate. Beyond that, individualize.

1. If the history suggests tension headache and the examination is normal, a treatment trial without further testing is reasonable.
2. Most patients with common or classic migraine deserve a computed tomography (CT) scan, or magnetic resonance imaging (MRI) at least once for reassurance that another process (e.g., arteriovenous malformation, mass lesion, infection) is not being overlooked.

3. CT or MRI is mandatory for a patient with ominous headache symptoms, or if there is a focal neurologic deficit or signs of increased intracranial pressure.

TREATMENT TIPS

Headache therapy consists first of altering environmental factors. Tapering off caffeinated beverages, avoiding precipitating foods and drink, getting regular exercise, altering changeable stressors, and performing relaxation exercises all have a place in therapy. Some patients develop a refractory headache disorder (transformed headache) caused by the regular use of headache medications, and must be "detoxified" before treatment can be effective.

Withdrawing caffeine may take months to show a benefit.

MIGRAINE HEADACHES

The following is indicated for treatment of acute migraine:

1. *Aspirin or acetaminophen* may help, although patients have usually already tried these.
2. *Caffeine* with aspirin, or acetaminophen, may be useful.
3. Therapy with *non-steroidal analgesics* (naproxen sodium, ibuprofen, or tolfenamic acid) may be effective.
4. The *triptans* are serotonin receptor agonists that act by constricting cranial vessels, and by inhibiting chemical mediators in peripheral branches of the trigeminal nerve. They vary in route of administration and time to maximum effect, duration of effect, and side effect profile.
   - *Sumatriptan* is a 5-hydroxytryptamine receptor agonist available in injection, nasal spray, and pill form and is effective in acute migraine.
   - *Zolmitriptan* is a serotonin agonist for acute headache therapy.
   - Other available triptans include almotriptan, eletriptan, frovatriptan, naratriptan, and rizatriptan.
5. *Fiorinal* (aspirin/butalbital/caffeine) often leads to an overuse syndrome. It has been banned in many countries due to its addictive potential.
6. *Anti-nauseants*, such as metochlopramide and chlorpromazine, may be helpful for nausea and headache (LOE = 1a). They may improve gastrointestinal motility, and facilitate absorption of more specific anti-migraine medications.

7. IV valproic acid may be useful in acute migraine (class A recommendation)

8. Intranasal dihydroergotamine may be effective. Other ergot derivatives, in general, are no longer used.

9. A *stratified care* model often is used, in which the patient takes different medications depending on the severity of the headache (LOE = 2b). This reduces treatment failures. It also ensures that appropriate medication is used early in the headache, when it is most likely to be effective.

10. Combination therapy may be more effective than individual agents alone.

11. Narcotics are seldom necessary, and are often counterproductive. They may block the effect of preventive medications (class C recommendation).

12. Remember, emphasize prevention over acute treatment. Acute medications for headache should not be used more than 2 days a week.

Prophylactic Medications

Prevention of migraines becomes important when there are three or more severe migraine headaches per month, and if there are less frequent but protracted attacks that interfere with function.

1. *Tricyclic antidepressants* (TCAs), such as amitriptyline and nortriptyline, are useful in migraine prophylaxis, especially with coexisting depression and tension-type headaches. Selective serotonin reuptake inhibitors are not as effective as TCAs in migraine prophylaxis, and may lead to serotonin syndrome when used with triptans (class A recommendation).

2. The *anti-epileptic medication*, valproic acid, is effective in migraine prophylaxis, although careful monitoring for idiosyncratic reactions is important. Topiramate also has more than one randomized trial showing its efficacy in migraine prophylaxis (class A recommendation).

3. Beta-blockers are an effective class of medications for migraine prophylaxis, with propranolol, atenolol, and nadolol being most effective (class A recommendation). Contraindications include asthma, diabetes, heart failure, heart block, depression, pregnancy, and Raynaud phenomenon.

4. *Calcium-channel blockers* are less useful than initially thought, and the results of trials of their use are disappointing. They may be worthwhile in patients with a prolonged aura, coexisting Raynaud syndrome or Prinzmetal angina, and in hemiplegic migraine.

5. Nonsteroidal medications (e.g., naproxen sodium), or estrogen supplementation may be particularly helpful in menstrual migraine therapy.
6. Other methods besides medications that have sufficient evidence to recommend them include butterbur root (class A), magnesium (class A), relaxation training (class A), and riboflavin (class A).

CLUSTER HEADACHES

1. Cluster headaches may be refractory to treatment once headache is established.
2. Oxygen, via a nonrebreather mask at a flow rate of 7 liters for 15 minutes, provides relief in approximately 70% of patients (class A recommendation).
3. Subcutaneous sumatriptan is very effective for the acute treatment of cluster headache. There does not appear to be tachyphylaxis, with daily use in cluster headache. It is not useful as a prophylactic medicine (class A recommendation). Intranasal sumatriptan is not as useful as subcutaneous.
4. Dihydroergotamine (DHE) in intravenous form is effective in cluster headache, but usually cannot be given in time by that route. Intranasal DHE is less effective, but helps some patients.
5. Zolmitriptan in 5- to 10-mg oral doses is effective in cluster headaches; although less so than subcutaneous sumatriptan, and with a moderate side effect profile.
6. Intranasal lidocaine 4% spray has a modest effect, and may be used in an adjunctive capacity in cluster headache.
7. Transitional prophylaxis during a cluster may be used to bridge to a more long-term prophylactic agent. Oral ergotamine tartrate 2 mg, or DHE 1 mg intramuscularly, can be used daily during a cluster with effective prevention of headaches. Both are contraindicated in patients with vascular disease, uncontrolled hypertension, or during pregnancy. A short course of steroids may be effective in transitional prophylaxis.
8. Maintenance prophylaxis is used for the expected duration of the cluster period. The following medications have shown efficacy in randomized placebo-controlled trials:
   - Verapamil.
   - Lithium carbonate.
   - Methysergide maleate.
   - Valproic acid.
   - Topiramate.

Each medication has its own set of side effects, which should be reviewed with the patient. Occipital nerve block with local anesthetic, and steroid injected around the nerve on the side of cluster, may cause headache relief. A tapering dose of steroids has also been shown to be effective in shortening a cluster period.

9. In chronic cluster headache, indomethacin and lithium may be effective.

TENSION HEADACHE

1. Aspirin, acetaminophen, and nonsteroidal anti-inflammatory drugs commonly are used.
2. Recurrent tension-type headaches may respond to lifestyle changes. Remember, some medications, or medical conditions (e.g., chronic renal failure) may make tension headache worse.
3. Make sure the patient does not have a medication overuse headache (discussed later in the chapter).
4. TCAs may be helpful in the prevention of chronic, tension-type headaches. Combined TCA therapy and stress management was superior to either alone (class A recommendation).
5. Neck massage, cervical pillow, relaxation exercises, and nontraditional therapies (e.g., acupuncture) may be helpful.
6. Regular physical exercise is helpful in most patients.

MEDICATION OVERUSE HEADACHE

Patients who frequently use analgesics, narcotics, caffeine, or the triptan medications may develop medication overuse headache or a "transformed" headache. The overuse causes drug-rebound headaches, leading to even more dependence on medication in a vicious cycle. In European headache centers, up to 10% of patients have this headache type. There are no specific guidelines for "how much is too much" medication. As a general rule, three or more acute headache medications for 5 days a week is excessive, with even less frequent dosing recommended for triptans and opiates. Many patients develop a progressively increasing attack frequency, with a reduction in headache-free periods. The character of the headaches may change to a more constant, tension-type headache pattern. The frequent use of headache medication interferes with the efficacy of prophylactic medications, and patients often report failing multiple preventive drugs. It is crucial to educate the patient about the syndrome, and develop a strategy for withdrawing the offending medications or drugs. This may be done in either an outpatient or inpatient setting. Once patients are no longer taking the acute medications, the headache character may revert to its original periodic pattern and respond to standard preventive therapies.

Notice the absence of information on "sinus headache." Although the public has been lead to believe that there is such an entity, most "sinus headache" is really migraine.

Acute sinusitis is unilateral, with focal tenderness, discharge, and often fever. It is treated with antibiotics and decongestants.

RARER HEADACHE SYNDROMES

1. SUNCT (short-lasting, unilateral, neuralgiform headache attacks with conjunctival injection, and tearing). More common in males over 50. Unilateral. Attacks are daytime, last for seconds to a few minutes, and patients can have a few attacks an hour. Autonomic features (watery eyes, nasal congestion, and sweaty forehead).

   May respond to corticosteroids, gabapentin, lamotrigine, and carbamazepine.

2. Chronic paroxysmal hemicrania (CPH): short-lasting pain, unilateral, usually orbital, attacks last 2 to 45 minutes, up to 5 attacks per day. There are also associated autonomic symptoms. May respond dramatically to indomethacin, dosed at 150 mg/day within a few days; otherwise tends to be refractory to other treatments.

Suggested Readings

Biondi D, Mendes P. Treatment of primary headache: cluster headache. In: *Standards of Care for Headache Diagnosis and Management.* Chicago: National Headache Foundation; 2004:59–74.

Chronicle E, Mulleners W. Anticonvulsant drugs for migraine prophylaxis (Cochrane Review). In: *The Cochrane Library.* Chichester, UK: Wiley; 2006: issue 2.

Goadsby PJ, Lipton RB. A review of paroxysmal hemicranias, SUNCT syndrome and other short-lasting headaches with autonomic feature, including new cases. *Brain.* 1997;120:193–209.

Institute for Clinical Systems Improvement (ICSI). *Diagnosis and Treatment of Headaches.* Bloomington, MN: ICSI; 2006.

Linde K, Rossnagel K. Propranolol for migraine prophylaxis (Cochrane Review). In: *The Cochrane Library*. Chichester, UK: Wiley; 2006: issue 2.

Lipton RB, Scher AL, Kolodner K. Migraine in the United States: epidemiology and patterns of health care use. *Neurology*. 2002;58:885–894.

Moja PL, Cusi C, Sterzi RR, et al. Selective serotonin re-uptake inhibitors for preventing migraine and tension-type headaches (Cochrane Review). In: *The Cochrane Library*. Chichester, UK: Wiley; 2006: issue 2.

Schreiber CP, Hutchinson S, Webster CF, et al. Prevalence of migraine in patients with a history of self-reported or physician-diagnosed "sinus" headache. *Arch Int Med*. 2004;164:1769–1772.

U.S. Headache Consortium. *Guidelines for Headache Management*. www.ahsnet.org/guidelines.php.

19 Dementia

CASE

An 82-year-old retired schoolteacher has had increasing problems functioning at home. She stopped driving a year ago, after she became lost on the way home from church. Nine months ago, her daughter took over paying the bills and grocery shopping, when she realized her mother could no longer balance her checkbook or make a shopping list. Her neurologic examination is unremarkable, except for a mini-mental status examination score of 16 out of a possible score of 30.

Diagnosis

Probable senile dementia of the Alzheimer type.

WHAT IS THE NATURE OF DEMENTIA?

Dementia is a loss of intellectual ability that interferes with a person's ability to function at work or in a social situation. It is chronic, developing over months and years. It affects multiple components of cognition such as judgment, language, initiative, spatial abilities, and memory. There are many causes of dementia, the most common being Alzheimer disease (AD) and multi-infarct dementia (MID). Treatments for AD have become available, increasing the importance of establishing a diagnosis.

DIAGNOSING DEMENTIA

1. Obtain a careful history. A careful history from the family is essential. Never depend on the patient's account alone. **Patients with dementia may lack insight into their problems.**
2. When did problems first begin and how rapidly have they progressed? Include questions about working, driving, shopping,

doing the checkbook, and self-grooming. Specific examples of functional problems are very useful in diagnosis.

3. Is there a problem with language? Does the patient have trouble finding words, or does the patient use unusual words (paraphasic errors)? These suggest a dominant hemisphere language area abnormality.

4. Is there a change in personality (i.e., more irritable or more placid)? Is the patient impulsive in decisions, or in conversation with others? Such changes may be seen in frontal lobe dementias, as well as in later stages of AD.

5. Has the patient lost initiative (e.g., given up hobbies or suggesting where to go on weekends)? This is seen with frontal lobe disease.

6. Does the patient get lost in the house, or lose the car in a parking lot? This may suggest nondominant parietal lobe dysfunction.

7. Is the patient ataxic or incontinent? Normal pressure hydrocephalus (NPH) causes the triad of dementia, ataxia, and incontinence. Gait disorders may occur in other dementias.

8. Is there evidence of depression? In the elderly, depression may mimic dementia and respond to antidepressants.

9. Are there medications, toxins, or "sleeping pills" that could be compromising intellect? Substance abuse (e.g., alcohol) and medication toxicity frequently are under-diagnosed in the elderly. **Statins may occasionally cause memory disorders, and are commonly prescribed.**

10. Are there medical illnesses that may have an impact on cognition? Is the patient positive for the human immunodeficiency virus (HIV), which is a major cause of dementia in younger adults?

11. Is there a family history of dementia? Often, this may be underplayed by the family. Ask about "senility" or failing faculties in the elderly. **First-degree relatives of patients with Alzheimer disease have an increased lifetime risk of developing Alzheimer disease.**

12. Is there a history of stroke, hypertension, diabetes, or other vascular risk factors? These may point to multi-infarct dementia.

13. Are there concurrent parkinsonism, mental fluctuations, and formed visual hallucinations? Lewy body dementia has these features.

14. Is there progressive headache, or focal neurologic symptoms, to suggest a mass lesion?

DEFINE THE MENTAL STATUS

The mental status is a bedside evaluation of cognitive function. Obviously this is only one measure of cognitive function. Extensive neuropsychiatric evaluation may be needed to precisely evaluate patients for deficits in different functional areas. There are readily available brief mental status tests (e.g., Folstein mini-mental status, short test of mental status, frontal assessment battery) that can be used as screening tools, and are quantitative. They can be used to quantify and track function over time. The definition of the mental status consists of the following components:

1. *State of consciousness.* If the patient is not fully awake, one should suspect a metabolic disorder, or a space-occupying lesion.

   Delirium is an acute, fluctuating mental state with prominent agitation, and hallucinations, as well as perceptual errors.

   Clues that the process may be delirium rather than dementia include:

   - Inattention.
   - Fluctuating symptoms.
   - Disturbances in sleep.
   - Prominent perceptual abnormalities.
   - Increased autonomic activity.

   Coma is when a patient has no conscious interaction with his or her environment.

   Stupor refers to a patient who interacts only when stimulated, but otherwise is indifferent to his or her environment.

   Obtundation is a term readily used by medical residents. However, it is one that lacks medical definition, and should be avoided.

   Observe what the patient does when left alone, and when you interact with the patient. Does the patient notice individuals in the room? Does he or she say hello and offer to shake hands? Check for attention by digit span (counting backwards from 100 by sevens; 20 by threes), or by having the patient recite the months of the year backwards. If a patient is inattentive, it will be difficult to interpret the rest of the mental status examination.

2. *Orientation* to place, person, and time. Is the patient able to tell the year, date, and day? Do they know where they are, the floor they are on, why they are there? Do they know who you are, or what you do?

3. *Aphasia* (see Chapter 4). Test naming, repetition, and evaluate spontaneous speech. Have the patient describe his or her occupation or favorite hobby in detail. Test his or her ability to read a newspaper, write when dictated to.

4. *Memory*. Can the patient remember a phone number of 7 digits? Can the patient repeat four objects immediately? Working memory or immediate recall is tested in this way. Retrieval of material after a few minutes is one measure of long-term memory (e.g., remembering four objects after doing another task).

5. *Calculation*. Have the patient do simple mathematical problems. Acalculia occurs in dominant hemisphere parietal disorders (angular gyrus).

6. *Abstraction*. Ask questions such as, "How are a ball and an orange alike?" or "What do a bathtub and the ocean have in common?"

7. *Judgment*. What would they do in the Denver airport with a dollar in their pocket (no cell phones, no debit, or credit cards)?

8. *Pictures*. How well can the patient interpret a picture in a magazine? Is there focus on one tiny part, and an inability to integrate it (asimultagnosia)? Does the patient have problems drawing or copying designs (constructional apraxia)?

9. *Mood and thought content*. Is the patient sad or inappropriately cheerful? Fearful or paranoid? Active or apathetic? Personally neat or sloppy? Is the patient's affect labile (does it vary from moment to moment)? Does the patient tell inappropriate jokes?

PERFORM CAREFUL GENERAL AND NEUROLOGIC EXAMINATIONS

1. For the general examination, is there evidence of liver, kidney, lung, heart, adrenal, or thyroid disease?

   Patients with general medical conditions may have cognitive dysfunction.

2. Is the blood pressure elevated? Is the heart rhythm regular?

   Hypertension and atrial fibrillation are markers for multi-infarct dementia.

3. Are there focal neurologic signs, papilledema, or upgoing toes? Are the reflexes brisk?

   Focal signs other than frontal release signs should signal a search for focal brain lesions such as stroke, tumor, infection, inflammation, and the like.

4. Check vision and hearing. Test for smell. Symptoms of dementia are made worse by sensory deprivation.

   Alzheimer disease and Parkinson disease may be preceded by a loss of smell.

5. Is the gait abnormal? Are there signs of parkinsonism?

   Gait disorders are common in dementia syndromes. They may precede the onset of frank dementia, and are a signal for evaluation in the elderly.

IS THERE A TUMOR?

1. Tumors presenting silently as dementia are often in the frontal lobes. Frontal lobe reflexes (suck, snout, grasp) may be present, and there is slowness in carrying out tasks. Smell may be impaired. Tumors occurring in other areas usually give focal signs. Seizures and gait disorders are common features of brain tumors.

2. Tumors obstructing the third or fourth ventricle may cause hydrocephalus and subsequent dementia, often with few focal signs. Intermittent exacerbation of symptoms is common, because of transient obstruction of the cerebrospinal fluid (CSF) pathway.

3. A normal computed tomography (CT) scan, with and without contrast, is usually sufficient to rule out tumor. Magnetic resonance imaging (MRI) is more sensitive than CT scan for brain tumor, especially for those located in the posterior fossa.

IS THERE NORMAL PRESSURE HYDROCEPHALUS (NPH)?

1. Consider NPH when mental deterioration occurs over 6 to 12 months, and there is an associated gait disorder and incontinence. Upgoing toes are common.

2. The pathophysiology of NPH is not well understood, but it involves inadequate absorption of CSF over the cerebral hemispheres, leading to hydrocephalus.

3. NPH may follow subarachnoid hemorrhage, meningitis, or head trauma, but it is often of unknown etiology.

4. No test is specific or diagnostic of NPH, although large ventricles in the absence of cortical atrophy are highly suggestive.

5. Improvement in gait after lumbar puncture (LP) and removal of CSF may be a helpful clue to the diagnosis; no tests predict the benefit of long-term shunting in this condition.

6. Complications after shunting are common, and include aspiration, infection, and subdural hematoma.

IS THERE A CHRONIC SUBDURAL HEMATOMA?

Sometimes after minor trauma, or trauma that is not remembered by the patient, slowly progressive subdural hematomas present with dementia. Headache, fluctuating symptoms, a gait abnormality, and relatively short-term progression are suggestive. Sometimes an isodense subdural will be missed on CT, so consider MRI. Do not perform a lumbar puncture (LP), because it is not diagnostic and may cause herniation.

VITAMIN B$_{12}$ DEFICIENCY

Altered cognitive function may be a consequence of vitamin B$_{12}$ deficiency. Onset may be insidious over months or years. Patients may not have the usual hematologic changes before neurologic symptoms. A borderline B$_{12}$ may be significant. Other confirmatory testing such as homocysteine level and methylmalonic acid level usually will be elevated if there is a true deficiency. Antiparietal cell antibodies, or intrinsic factor antibodies are usually positive in pernicious anemia. Look for associated paresthesias, and posterior and lateral column spinal cord signs (subacute combined degeneration; see Chapter 13).

METABOLIC DISEASES

Patients with dementia secondary to hepatic, renal, and endocrine diseases usually do not have a clear sensorium. In young patients with liver disease and dementia or depression, check for Wilson disease (ceruloplasmin and 24-hour urinary copper). Check for hypothyroidism, consider the possibility of hypoglycemia (e.g., in a patient with diabetes being treated with insulin), and Cushing disease.

INFECTIOUS DISEASES

Consider cerebrospinal fluid (CSF) examination in selected patients for tuberculosis, or fungal or carcinomatous meningitis. Patients with acquired immunodeficiency syndrome (AIDS) may develop an encephalopathy with behavioral changes and dementia (HIV-associated dementia). Syphilis serology is no longer routinely obtained unless:

1. The patient is at high risk (e.g., AIDS).
2. There are signs or symptoms suggesting syphilis.
3. The patient lives in an endemic area for syphilis.

DRUG AND TOXINS

Sleeping medication, anti-anxiety drugs, and alcohol are important causes of cognitive dysfunction in the elderly. Barbiturates and benzodiazepines may cause cognitive dysfunction. Oxybutynin and diphenhydramine may also cause cognitive impairment. Patients may not consider sleeping pills to be "medication," and may not list them on forms.

DEPRESSION

Depression may present as dementia in the elderly, and this condition sometimes is referred to as a "pseudodementia." Suggestive features include:

1. History of psychiatric disease.
2. Relatively brief duration of symptoms.
3. Vegetative symptoms of depression, including anorexia, weight loss, altered sleep pattern, decreased concentration, loss of energy, and psychomotor retardation.

Specific features of depression include :

1. Sadness.
2. Guilt.
3. Apathy.
4. Social withdrawal.
5. Episodes of weeping.
6. Suicidal ideas.

Pseudodementia has been shown to presage true dementia in some patients; therefore, treatment of the depression may be only part of the required therapy.

Although "treatable" causes of dementia may be found, it is rare that treatment completely reverses cognitive deficits in this population.

DIAGNOSTIC WORKUP FOR DEMENTIA

A basic screen for dementia should include a complete blood count, urinalysis, measurement of electrolyte, calcium, blood urea nitrogen, vitamin B_{12}, sedimentation rate, liver function tests, thyroid function tests, serologic tests for syphilis (in endemic areas), HIV testing (where appropriate), drug levels (where appropriate), electrocardiogram, chest radiograph, CT scan or MRI of the brain, lumbar puncture (LP) if chronic meningitis or opportunistic infection is suspected, and neuropsychologic testing (where appropriate). With a careful history, physical examination, and the preceding studies, the etiology of dementia should become clear in most cases. If the diagnosis remains uncertain, other studies, such as arteriography or brain biopsy, may be necessary.

ALZHEIMER DISEASE AND OTHER DEMENTIAS

Alzheimer Disease

The most common cause of dementia is Alzheimer disease (AD). The following features are characteristic of the disease:

1. Progression is slow, over years, without a stepwise change.
2. Gradually developing forgetfulness is the key feature, eventually accompanied by problems with other cognitive tasks. Day-to-day events, names, places, and directions to familiar sites all may be forgotten. Language problems, with difficulty finding certain words, may occur. Problems with mathematics are common, usually manifested with using the checkbook. Visuospatial problems occur (e.g., analyzing a picture, difficulty drawing or copying figures, or difficulty figuring out how mechanical appliances work). Alertness is preserved until late stages. Wandering is a frequent problem.
3. The patient is often brought to the physician by the family, and is unaware that there is a problem (lack of insight).
4. There are usually no neurologic signs apart from the dementia; toes are usually downgoing, and the patient is generally sociable and neat in the early stages. A grasp or snout response may be present. Later, personality change is frequent. There is sometimes visual agnosia (the ability to see, but not recognize, objects) and motor apraxia (inability to perform certain stereotyped motor tasks in the absence of paralysis). At advanced stages, seizures may occur in about 15% of patients.

5. A substantial subset of patients with AD develops extrapyramidal signs late in the disease.

6. CT or MRI shows nonspecific findings of atrophy and ventricular dilatation. Electroencephalogram (EEG) shows slowing most prominently in the temporal regions, and irregular background, but these changes are nonspecific, and EEG is generally not necessary.

7. The pathology consists of neuronal loss, deposition of amyloid plaques, neurofibrillary tangles, and secondary inflammatory changes. Research into deposition of these substances and the genetics of AD may offer effective treatment in the future.

8. There is a link between Alzheimer disease and apolipoprotein E (ApoE). Testing for this has not been very helpful in diagnosis (neither rules in nor rules out the diagnosis).

9. Education and continuing mental stimulation delay cognitive impairment. Physical activity is beneficial for reducing cognitive impairment and reducing the risk of dementia in persons age 65 and older.

10. For *treatment*, cholinesterase inhibitors may provide temporary improvement or stabilization of the disease. Donepezil is a cholinesterase inhibitor that is well tolerated, and is used for symptomatic treatment of Alzheimer disease. Other cholinesterase inhibitors with modest efficacy include rivastigmine and galantamine. Gastrointestinal side effects are the most common adverse events with this class of medication. Ginkgo biloba, a plant extract, has a modest effect on cognitive function in AD. Memantine is an NMDA receptor antagonist that is helpful in moderate AD. The extent of benefit of these medications is modest at best.

11. Drugs to modify disruptive behavior include neuroleptics, anxiolytics, and antidepressants. These drugs should be used cautiously, because patients in this age group often have adverse responses to these medications. For antidepressants, selective serotonin reuptake inhibitor medications are preferred because of their low incidence of adverse side effects in the elderly. Trazodone may be used if there is disordered nighttime sleep. Buspirone may be effective for anxiety in patients with Alzheimer disease. **Atypical antipsychotics are not routinely recommended. They are associated with an increase in cerebrovascular events, as well as increased mortality (level 1a evidence).**

    Note: A distinction needs to be made between minimal cognitive impairment (MCI), and dementia. MCI is a condition in which patients forget more readily than in the past, but in which virtually all other cognitive functions are intact.

About 10% to 20% of such patients go on to having a dement-ing disorder (usually Alzheimer disease), but many may not progress at all.

Multi-Infarct Dementia

Multi-infarct dementia (MID) refers to dementia associated with multiple infarctions. MID is sometimes difficult to separate clini-cally from Alzheimer disease, and may be part of a "mixed" demen-tia (i.e., both AD and MID are present). Suggestive features include:

1. Vascular risk factors.
2. History of strokes.
3. A stepwise progression.
4. Focal neurologic signs.
5. Pseudobulbar palsy.
6. MRI or CT changes of significant multifocal ischemic disease.

Multi-infarct dementia may occur in patients treated inade-quately for hypertension, and is therefore potentially preventable. Furthermore, treatment of hypertension may prevent progression. Cholinesterase inhibitors may be helpful in the cognitive impair-ment of some patients with MID.

Creutzfeldt–Jakob Disease

Creutzfeldt–Jakob disease (CJD) is a rare, rapidly progressive dis-order caused by a proteinaceous infectious agent (prion). The prion appears to be an abnormal conformation of a naturally occurring protein. A profound dementia, ataxia, and myoclonic jerks are characteristic, and often progress over weeks. Visual loss and motor neuron changes may occur. EEG may show periodic sharp and slow waves that assist in the diagnosis. Pathologically, the brain shows spongiform changes with vacuoles. MRI may show characteristic T2 image changes in the striatum in CJD. A spinal fluid assay for the 14-3-3 brain protein supports the diag-nosis if positive, but it is not specific for CJD and is positive in other neurodegenerative disorders. Death occurs in a few weeks to several months, and there is no effective treatment.

Pick Disease

Pick disease (frontotemporal dementia) resembles Alzheimer dis-ease clinically, but is quite rare and pathologically distinct. Personality changes, altered judgment, apathy, and prominent frontal release signs are more marked than in AD. Pathologically, Pick disease affects frontal and temporal lobes more than parietal lobes. Many cases of primary progressive aphasia have Pick type pathology at autopsy. Pick disease is considered one of the frontotemporal dementias.

Huntington Disease

Huntington disease presents as an insidious intellectual decline associated with psychiatric symptoms and chorea. Dementia, personality changes, and emotional disorder may precede the chorea. Inheritance is autosomal dominant, and involves a genetic abnormality on the short arm of chromosome 4. An excess of a trinucleotide repeat (CAG) at the Huntington gene locus confers the disease, and an increased number of repeats is associated with earlier onset of the disease. Family history is usually positive, but must be diligently explored. Genetic testing and counseling are available. Genetic testing should not be obtained without psychological support to the patient and family by knowledgeable care providers.

Lewy Body Dementia

Lewy body dementia is a common cause of dementia. In addition to dementia, characteristic clinical features include day-to-day fluctuations in the patient's cognitive or functional abilities, visual hallucinations, and prominent extrapyramidal signs. Extreme sensitivity to neuroleptic medications is characteristic. There are no specific diagnostic tests. Pathologically, the disease is characterized by Lewy bodies (eosinophilic cytoplasmic inclusions in neurons) in the cortex and subcortex. The patient may respond to cholinesterase inhibitors, but tends to be less responsive to dopaminergic agents than are patients with Parkinson disease.

Cortocobasal Degeneration with Neuronal Achromasia

Cortocobasal degeneration with neuronal achromasia is a rare disorder in which patients have a progressive dementia, which may be marked by a striking lateralization of findings. They may have a neglect syndrome, or constructional apraxia. They often have an alien hand or dystonic posturing of the hand contralateral to the major hemispheric involvement. There are neuronal pathologic inclusions unique to this entity. There are no specific treatments.

Suggested Readings

Burnett MG, Sonnad SS, Stein SC. Screening tests for normal-pressure hydrocephalus: sensitivity, specificity, and cost. *J Neurosurg*. 2006;105:823–829.

Knight R. Creutzfeldt-Jakob disease: a rare cause of dementia in elderly persons. *Clin Infect Dis*. 2006;43:340–346.

Knopman DS, Petersen RC, Cha RH, et al. Incidence and causes of nondegenerative nonvascular dementia: a population-based study. *Arch Neurol*. 2006;63:218–221.

Larson EB, Wang L, Bowen JD, et al. Exercise is associated with reduced risk for incident dementia among persons 65 years of age or older. *Ann Int Med*. 2006;144:73–81.

Samanta MK, Wilson B, Santhi K, et al. Alzheimer disease and its management: a review. *Am J Ther*. 2006;13:516–526.

Schneider LS, Dagerman KS, Insel P. Risk of death with atypical antipsychotic drug treatment for dementia: meta-analysis of randomized placebo-controlled trials. *JAMA*. 2005;294:1934–1943.

Walker FO. Huntington's disease. *Lancet*. 2007;369:218–228.

Weisman D, McKeith I. Dementia with Lewy bodies. *Semin Neurol*. 2007;27:42–47.

20 Seizures and Epilepsy

CASE

A 17-year-old senior in high school with no history of prenatal injury, febrile convulsions, head injury, or meningitis is being treated with valproic acid for seizures, and has been seizure free for 1 year. At age 13, he had the first of three generalized tonic-clonic seizures. At age 15, he noticed that his body would jerk for a few minutes after awakening, and on one occasion this was followed by a convulsion. At age 16, he was noticed to stare from time to time in school. His electroencephalogram (EEG) shows generalized spike-and-wave activity.

Diagnosis

Juvenile myoclonic epilepsy with associated absence seizures.

A seizure reflects a transient neurologic event caused by the sudden abnormal discharge of a group of cerebral neurons. In general, seizures are a symptom of underlying brain disease—not a diagnosis. Epilepsy is the condition of repeated spontaneous and unprovoked seizures. Epilepsy has a variety of causes, both genetically determined and acquired.

Epilepsy means a state of recurring, unprecipitated seizures, and has no other implications.

TYPES OF SEIZURES

Seizures are categorized into two major types, depending on the presumed source: partial (focal) seizures or generalized seizures (Table 20.1).

In *partial (focal) seizures*, the initial discharge comes from a specific part of the brain. Such patients have symptoms that depend on the area of cortex involved. Thus, patients whose seizures begin with their right hand shaking or with an aura of smelling "burned candy" have a partial seizure disorder, attributable to a lesion in the frontal or temporal lobe, respectively. Partial

■ TABLE 20.1. Classification of Seizures

Partial (Focal)	Generalized
Simple partial	Absence
Complex partial	Myoclonic, tonic, atonic, etc.
Tonic-clonic (secondary)	Tonic-clonic (primary)

seizures with impairment of consciousness are known as complex partial seizures. Remember, a seizure can begin focally and then generalize. This may happen so quickly that it is impossible to see the focality clinically, and the patient can recall no aura. Nonetheless, the electroencephalogram (EEG) usually shows the focality, and historical clues (brain tumor, arteriovenous malformation [AVM]) may suggest a focal origin. Partial seizure disorders are usually secondary to local pathology (e.g., trauma, tumor, vascular lesions, or congenital abnormalities).

It is important to recognize that partial complex seizures may be manifest only by unusual and paroxysmal changes in behavior, without loss of consciousness or convulsive motor activity. This is especially true in the elderly, in which the incidence of epilepsy is increasing dramatically, and in which the manifestations of seizures can be unusual.

In *generalized seizures*, there are no focal sites of seizure origin. There is no aura, and there are no focal features during the seizure. Examples of generalized seizures include absence seizures (previously called petit mal) and idiopathic tonic-clonic seizures (previously called grand mal). A tonic-clonic seizure is a major motor seizure involving all extremities, and having tonic (stiffening) and clonic (rhythmic jerking) movements. Myoclonic jerks (rapid individual muscle movements) also may be seen in primary generalized epilepsy, often as a syndrome in teenage years, combined with absence seizures and rare tonic-clonic seizures (juvenile myoclonic epilepsy of Janz).

Note: Seizures may follow unusual stress ("precipitated convulsions") and are not considered epilepsy.

Precipitated convulsions do not equal epilepsy.

Establish whether the seizure disorder is focal or generalized.

HISTORY

Is there a history of unusual behavior, with or without loss of consciousness, which is not explained by other medical diagnoses?

Does the patient remember the event? Is there any retrograde amnesia? Is there confusion after the event?

1. Exactly how did the seizure start? Find a witness. Did the head and eyes turn? Were there other focal features? Was there an aura?
2. At what age did the seizures begin? This is important. Primary generalized seizures rarely begin before age 3 years or after age 18. "Absence seizures" that begin during adulthood, are usually complex partial seizures of temporal lobe origin.
3. Is there a family history of seizures? This may be present in both types, but is more characteristic of generalized seizure disorders.
4. Was there focal trauma at birth, or during an accident (head trauma)? Is there a history of a previous neurologic insult (e.g., stroke, encephalitis, meningitis)?
5. Does the patient have abdominal pains, nausea, dizziness, behavioral disturbances, or automatisms (frequent features of temporal lobe epilepsy)? Are there déjà vu phenomena (vivid memories of prior experiences)? Does the patient smell an odd smell for a few moments (a common symptom of seizures from the mesial temporal lobe)?
6. Have there been brief staring spells not followed by post-ictal confusion, or fatigue (absence seizures)?

EXAMINATION

1. Look for post-ictal paralysis (Todd paralysis) by checking for asymmetry of reflexes, hemiparesis, an upgoing toe, or hemi-paretic posturing of a leg.
2. Look for asymmetry of fingernail, toe, and limb size (a clue to early damage to the contralateral hemisphere).
3. Absence seizures (a primary generalized seizure of childhood) can be precipitated by hyperventilation. Have the patient breathe deeply for 5 minutes, and watch for a brief, transient cessation of activity and "glassy stare."
4. Examine the skin carefully. Neurocutaneous disorders such as neurofibromatosis, tuberous sclerosis, and Sturge–Weber disease may present with seizures.

LABORATORY AIDS IN DIAGNOSIS

1. In addition to baseline laboratory studies (including glucose, blood urea nitrogen, calcium, sodium), perform an EEG,

a magnetic resonance imaging (MRI) scan, or computed tomography (CT) scan for any unexplained first seizure. An MRI is more sensitive than a CT scan in locating the etiology in focal seizures.

2. Obtain a sleep-deprived EEG if a focal seizure disorder is suspected. Frequently, it will bring out the spike focus. In some cases, the spike focus can be seen only with special (e.g., anterior temporal or sphenoidal) EEG leads.

3. MRI is accurate in detecting small tumors, focal gliosis, cortical dysgenesis, and mesial temporal sclerosis, all of which may cause partial seizures. Coronal thin slices through the temporal lobes using fluid-attenuation inversion recovery (FLAIR) sequences increase the yield of MRI in focal epilepsies.

Many patients with epilepsy do not have structural lesions on imaging. This in no way stands against the diagnosis of epilepsy.

WHAT ETIOLOGIC FACTORS ARE INVOLVED?

Drug withdrawal (from alcohol, barbiturates, and other sedatives) is a common cause of seizures in adults. Alcohol withdrawal seizures occur 12 to 48 hours after the cessation of drinking (see Chapter 27). Alcoholics with post-traumatic epilepsy secondary to frequent falls may have an exacerbation of seizures when intoxicated.

Exacerbation of a known seizure disorder is common. Persons with a controlled seizure disorder, who come to the hospital because of a recurrence, usually have:

1. Not been taking their medication (draw blood level).
2. Been drinking.
3. An intercurrent infection.

Change in lifestyle, emotional stress, menses, or sleep deprivation also may exacerbate seizures. Temporarily increase the medication, if seizures occur during a period of intercurrent infection. Reevaluate anyone with a well-controlled seizure disorder that worsens with no apparent cause. More than half of the cases of *post-traumatic epilepsy* develop during the first year after injury, and more than 80% develop by 4 years. There occasionally are delayed cases. Penetrating injuries of the dura, cerebral hemorrhage and contusion, brain infection, focal neurologic signs, and prolonged coma all increase the risk of epilepsy. A seizure immediately after head injury is not a specific risk factor for epilepsy, but seizures within the first week increase that risk.

Subdural hematoma can be associated with seizures and must be considered in an alcoholic with new onset of seizures.

Etiology as related to *age of onset* is as follows:

- Infancy and childhood: birth injury, congenital malformations, infections, trauma, metabolic disorders, genetic, idiopathic.
- Adolescence: idiopathic, genetic, trauma, drug-related.
- Young adult: trauma, alcohol, neoplasm, drug-related, arterio-venous malformation (AVM).
- Middle age: neoplasm, alcohol, vascular disease, trauma, AVM.
- Late life (older than age 65 years): vascular disease, neoplasm, associated with dementia.

Note: Idiopathic or primary generalized epilepsy usually is apparent by age 18. Seizures beginning after age 18 usually are caused by a focal process, metabolic derangement, or withdrawal state. Neoplasm is of prime concern during all of adult life. After age 65 years, vascular disease (stroke) is the most common cause of a first seizure.

Genetic etiologies for seizures are important in infants and young adults. Epilepsies previously labeled idiopathic now are known to be genetic. Genetic transmission of seizures can be autosomal dominant, autosomal recessive, or mitochondrial. Examples of genetic epilepsies include childhood absence epilepsy and juvenile myoclonic epilepsy.

SEIZURES VERSUS SYNCOPE

Neurologists are frequently called to evaluate patients who have lost consciousness suddenly to decide if this is "seizure versus syncope." In fact, these are usually readily distinguished by the clinical story (Table 20.2). Syncope patients often have a characteristic prodrome, where they feel faint, have blurry vision, sweatiness, and a sense that "they are going to pass out." In contrast, these are uncommon in seizure, and the aura of seizure is usually a specific neurologic symptom such as a smell, a sense of déjà vu, or a rising sensation. Syncope lasts seconds, whereas a seizure usually lasts a couple of minutes. A common source of confusion is patients with convulsive syncope. A few brief jerks with syncope are common, though more prolonged convulsive movements are uncommon in syncope.

Convulsive syncope is commonly confused with seizure.

A key question to ask is where did the patient wake up? Most patients with seizures awaken in the ambulance, whereas patients

■ TABLE 20.2. Differentiating Seizure Versus Syncope

Clinical Symptom/Sign	Syncope	Seizure
Prodromal symptoms	Nausea, faintness, blurred vision, sweating, muffled hearing	Aura (visual, auditory, gustatory, olfactory, déjà vu, etc.)
Duration	Seconds	1–2 minutes
Convulsive movements	Occasionally, a few tonic jerks	More prolonged tonic jerking
Awakens where?	Right where they fall	Later, in the ambulance
Tongue biting	No	Yes
Incontinence	No	Yes
Confusion after the event?	No	Yes

with syncope awaken right where they went down. Tongue biting is rare in syncope, as is incontinence. Finally, patients with syncope awaken immediately aware of their surroundings, whereas those with seizure are usually confused.

SUDDEN UNEXPECTED DEATH IN EPILEPSY

Sudden unexpected death in epilepsy (SUDEP) occurs approximately in 1 out of 300 patients with epilepsy per year in adulthood. These deaths do not occur in the context of trauma, drowning, or status epilepticus. SUDEP is common with severe epilepsy, and in patients who have poorly controlled epilepsy. SUDEP occurs more commonly in males than females, and usually in the young adult years. SUDEP may occur with changes in seizure medications, or with poor compliance with antiepileptic drugs (AEDs).

TREATMENT TIPS

Drugs for Partial Seizure Disorders

In general, there is no benefit in treatment for the first seizure, as recurrence rate is unclear in this population. Treatment is initiated with a single agent. Patients who fail the first agent are less likely to be completely controlled with subsequent medications. Traditional drugs used for partial seizures include carbamazepine and phenytoin.

Oxcarbazepine and lamotrigine can be used in monotherapy for partial seizures, but have a higher cost than carbamazepine. As a rule, do not use two drugs unless one drug in adequate dosage (check blood levels) does not control the seizures.

Newer drugs such as gabapentin, levetiracetam, lamotrigine, tiagabine, topiramate, and zonisamide are available as add-on medications for the treatment of complex partial seizures, but have a higher cost than other AEDs. Many of these medications are used as monotherapy, despite being primarily tested as add-on therapy in clinical trials. Many of the newer AEDs are better tolerated and have different side effect profiles than the older drugs. For example, many do not induce liver enzymes, and therefore will not interfere with oral contraceptive medication or warfarin. It is best to tailor the choice of first drug to the patient (Table 20.3).

Drugs for Primary Generalized Seizure Disorders

Valproic acid, carbamazepine, and phenytoin are first-line medications for primary generalized seizures. Alternatives include lamotrigine, levetiracetam, and topiramate. Ethosuximide may be used alone for absence seizures, but only if there are no associated tonic-clonic seizures (it has no activity against these). Valproic acid is useful in absence seizures, especially when there are associated tonic-clonic seizures.

CONVULSIVE STATUS EPILEPTICUS

Convulsive status epilepticus has been defined as continuous seizure activity for 30 minutes, or recurrent seizures for 30 minutes without resumption of consciousness. Evidence suggests that even shorter periods of continuous seizures can be deleterious to the brain, and the definition of "status epilepticus" is undergoing some revision. Convulsive status epilepticus, whatever its definition, remains a true medical emergency.

1. Maintain airway, administer O_2, prevent aspiration, and maintain blood pressure (ABCs). While doing so, obtain a brief history from family or friends, and perform a brief examination (e.g., is the patient a known epileptic who stopped taking medication or developed an infection?).
2. Draw blood to check glucose, electrolytes, calcium, magnesium, complete blood count, and toxic screens. Check antiepileptic drug (AED) levels if appropriate. Check oxygenation. Start an

TABLE 20.3. Common Medications Used in Epilepsy

Medication	Daily Starting Dose	Type of Epilepsy	Side Effects	Relative Cost	Efficacy
Carbamazepine	200–600 mg	G, PS	Ataxia, h, hem, r, hyponatremia	$$	***
Phenytoin	200–400 mg	G, PS	r, h, hem, many others	$	***
Valproic acid	15 mg/kg/day	G, PS, A, M	h, hem, pancreatitis	$$	***
Oxcarbazepine	600–1200 mg	G, PS	Like carbamazepine	$$$	***
Gabapentin	300–900 mg	PS (add on)	Fatigue, weight gain	$$$$	**
Lamotrigine	12.5–25 mg	G, PS, A, M	Rash, severe	$$$$	***
Topiramate	25 mg	G, PS (add on)	Cognitive, dizziness	$$$$	***
Levetiracetam	1000 mg	G, PS (add on)	Irritability	$$$$	***

G, generalized seizures; PS, partial seizures; A, absence seizures; M, myoclonic; h, hepatic; hem, hematologic; r, rash.

intravenous (IV) line, and administer 100 mg thiamine followed by 50 mL of 50% glucose.

3. Administer either 4 mg lorazepam IV push, or 10 mg of diazepam IV push. Either drug may cause respiratory arrest, especially in patients who previously have been administered barbiturates, and thus should be used cautiously. These drugs stop seizures, but have a relatively short duration of action, and need to be followed by a second AED for longer-term control. If seizures continue for more than 10 minutes, an additional dose of either medication can be given.

4. Phenytoin or fos-phenytoin may be used for status epilepticus (phenytoin or phenytoin equivalents 15 to 18 mg/kg intravenously over 30 to 45 minutes). Either may be increased to 30 mg/kg if seizures continue. Hypotension can occur if phenytoin is given too quickly. Thus, do not administer phenytoin faster than 50 mg/minute, and have blood pressure and electrocardiogram monitored periodically during IV administration.

   Fos-phenytoin may be administered up to 150 mg/minute, but is metabolized to phenytoin, so that the onset of action is equivalent to that of phenytoin.

   Use phenytoin cautiously in patients with heart disease. In those with conduction defects, phenytoin is relatively contraindicated. For administration, phenytoin is given intravenously in normal saline; it will precipitate in dextrose solutions.

   Fos-phenytoin is a dilantin prodrug. It may be given intramuscularly. It appears to have less cardiotoxicity. It must be converted into phenytoin to be active; thus, its mode of action is similar to that of phenytoin. Phlebitis is more common with phenytoin than with fos-phenytoin.

5. Refractory status epilepticus has a high mortality. Medications that have been tried in small series include pentobarbital, high-dose phenobarbital, midazolam infusions, propofol infusions, and other medications, such as ketamine.

   Treatment of refractory status requires intubation for respiratory insufficiency and airway control, careful intensive care unit monitoring, preferably continuous EEG monitoring, and neurologic consultation. The EEG in these cases is titrated to a burst-suppression pattern (i.e., an anesthetic level of anesthesia). Vasopressors may be necessary.

6. When it proves difficult to control status epilepticus, there is often an underlying metabolic disorder (e.g., hyponatremia, hypoglycemia) or structural lesion (e.g., subdural, meningitis). Imaging and lumbar puncture (LP) should be considered in this setting.

7. The most likely etiology of status epilepticus if there is no history of seizures is stroke, tumor, or trauma. If there is a history of seizures, an intercurrent illness or noncompliance with medication is usually responsible.

Note: Mortality from status epilepticus increases dramatically with duration of status. Early effective treatment is critical.

THERAPEUTIC AGENTS

Phenytoin (Dilantin)

The average adult dose is 300 to 400 mg/day. Therapeutic blood levels are 10 to 20 mg/mL. Levels should be monitored in any patient who has not achieved good seizure control by taking phenytoin or other anticonvulsant medications. Some patients require a level outside the standard therapeutic range for optimal control. It may be useful to obtain a level when the patient is doing well, to assess an optimal dose for that patient.

Administered orally, it may take 3 to 5 days to achieve a steady state; IV administration in adequate doses gives therapeutic levels within an hour. Patients also may be given loading doses orally (e.g., 500 mg initially, followed by 300 mg 2 hours later, and 200 to 400 mg 2 hours later, followed by daily maintenance doses).

Intramuscular phenytoin is not absorbed evenly, causes muscle necrosis, and should be avoided. Fos-phenytoin may be given intravenously or intramuscularly. Nystagmus on lateral gaze is a good clinical sign that the patient is taking the medication. Ataxia of gait and lethargy are common manifestations of toxicity. Irritability and diplopia are other dose-related symptoms. Phenytoin is metabolized by the liver, so one usually can give regular doses to patients who have renal disease or are in renal failure. It is of value to check the level of free (unbound, active) phenytoin in these patients, and in pregnant patients taking phenytoin. A morbilliform rash occurs in approximately 4% of patients. If this occurs, it is best to stop the phenytoin use and choose an alternate anticonvulsant. Other side effects include hirsutism, gingival hypertrophy, megaloblastic anemia, osteomalacia, lymphadenopathy, and lupus-like syndrome. A teratogenic effect of phenytoin has been reported. With long-term use, cerebellar degeneration or a polyneuropathy may occur. IV phenytoin may cause phlebitis, but IV fos-phenytoin does not. Warfarin and isoniazid enhance the action of phenytoin, and INR may be altered by phenytoin in patients on warfarin. Chronic administration of barbiturates may decrease blood phenytoin levels. Patients taking phenytoin may have factitiously low thyroid function test levels. Phenytoin levels may increase suddenly when its receptor sites are saturated.

Thus, when a patient whose seizures are not yet controlled has a blood level in the therapeutic range, use 30-mg capsules to titrate the dose, or alternate 300 and 400 mg daily.

Despite its long-standing role in epilepsy, phenytoin is being used less and less, primarily because of its side effect profile and its complex pharmacology.

Carbamazepine

The carbamazepine dosage in adults is 600 to 1,200 mg/day in three divided doses. Long-acting forms (Tegretol-XR or Carbatrol) allow for twice-a-day dosing. A gradual dose escalation avoids many of the problems of initiating carbamazepine, including gastrointestinal upset, and those related to the delayed induction of hepatic enzymes. Therapeutic blood levels are 4 to 12 mg/mL.

Toxic side effects include:

1. Leukopenia.
2. Thrombocytopenia.
3. Hepatic dysfunction.
4. Hyponatremia.

Hyponatremia may be renally mediated. Dose-related side effects include sedation, ataxia, diplopia, and blurred vision. Carbamazepine is effective for focally originating seizures (drug of choice) and tonic-clonic seizures. Occasionally, carbamazepine may exacerbate absence seizures in patients being treated for primary generalized tonic-clonic seizures. Neural tube defects are reported in 1% of children born to mothers who are taking carbamazepine. Watch for a dramatic increase in carbamazepine levels, with concurrent use of erythromycin or propoxyphene, which block hepatic metabolism of this medication.

Valproic Acid

The initial dose is 15 mg/kg. Titration up to 60 mg/kg is necessary in some cases. Therapeutic blood levels are 50 to 100 mg/mL, although blood levels may correlate poorly with clinical response. Valproic acid is most effective in absence, myoclonic, and akinetic seizures and primary generalized epilepsies.

Toxic effects include:

1. Gastrointestinal disturbances and sedation (especially if the dose is built up rapidly).
2. Ataxia.
3. Liver dysfunction.
4. Thrombocytopenia.
5. Pancreatitis.

Hair loss, weight gain, and tremor are noticeable side effects in some patients. Hepatic failure may be seen in children younger than age 2 years who are treated with polypharmacy; it is rare in adults. Teratogenic effects with neural tube defects occur in 1% to 2% of children born to mothers taking valproic acid. Thus, this drug should be avoided in pregnant women, if possible. Interactions with other anticonvulsant medications include increased phenobarbital levels and increased free phenytoin levels.

Oxcarbazepine

Oxcarbazepine is closely related to carbamazepine, and has been used in Europe since the early 1990s. It may be used as monotherapy for partial and secondarily generalized seizures. It may aggravate absence or myoclonic seizures.

The usual total adult dose is 1,200 to 2,400 mg/day, with the drug given twice a day. Adverse effects are similar to carbamazepine. Leukopenia occurs less frequently than with carbamazepine. Hyponatremia may occur more commonly. It is generally well tolerated, with a favorable side effect profile.

Gabapentin

For dosage, begin with 300 mg the first day, increasing to 900 mg/day in three divided doses. Some patients are treated with up to 5,400 mg/day for refractory seizures. Gabapentin is used primarily as an add-on medication for partial seizures, although it has been shown to be effective in monotherapy.

Dose-related side effects include dizziness, somnolence, and fatigue. Gabapentin is not metabolized significantly, remains unbound, and has virtually no interactions with other medications. It is excreted by the kidney and has an excellent safety profile. Gabapentin has modest efficacy in the treatment of partial seizures. Weight gain is occasionally seen as a side effect.

Lamotrigine

Very gradually titrate, over weeks, to a dose of 200 to 600 mg/day in two divided doses. A lower dose and slower titration is used in patients taking valproic acid. Lamotrigine is an effective medication for partial and generalized seizures, and may be used as an add-on drug for partial epilepsies. It has a broad spectrum of efficacy for epilepsy.

Side effects include skin rash, somnolence, and dizziness. Hypersensitivity rash is most common, with rapid titration, and rare cases of Stevens–Johnson syndrome being reported. **Patients must be counseled to stop lamotrigine *immediately* if rash occurs.** The half-life is 12 hours with enzyme-inducing medications, 24 hours with monotherapy, and 48 to 72 hours with concomitant valproic acid.

Lamotrigine may worsen myoclonic seizures.

Felbamate

Aplastic anemia and hepatic failure have made felbamate a medication to be used only by neurologists experienced with its toxicity; usually after failure of other seizure medication. It is approved for treatment of refractory partial epilepsy and for patients with Lennox–Gastaut syndrome. It is used alone or in combination with other antiepileptic drugs (AEDs).

Tiagabine

Tiagabine is used as an add-on medication for partial seizures. Tiagabine is generally well tolerated. Adverse effects include dizziness, asthenia, nervousness, tremor, depressed mood, and emotional lability. Its efficacy is relatively modest.

Topiramate

Topiramate is an add-on medication for partial seizures and secondary generalized seizures. Significant side effects include somnolence, blurred vision, and ataxia. Effective doses are between 200 and 400 mg/day using b.i.d. dosing.

Side effects include fatigue, gastrointestinal upset, dizziness, impaired thinking, and irritability. Renal calculi occur in 1% to 3% of patients; thus, adequate fluid intake should be encouraged. Other less common but important side effects include acute glaucoma and metabolic acidosis.

Levetiracetam

Levetiracetam is approved as an add-on medication for partial seizures. It is also approved as add-on medication for primary generalized epilepsy and myoclonic epilepsy in children age 12 or older.

Usual dosages are 1,000 to 3,000 mg/day in b.i.d. dosing.

Side effects include somnolence, irritability, asthenia, and dizziness. Drug interactions are limited. Safety appears to be excellent with this medication, and efficacy is good. Effective dosage in generalized seizures appears to be 3,000 mg/day.

Zonisamide

Zonisamide is approved as an add-on medication for partial seizures in patients who are 12 years or older. It also may be effective in generalized seizures.

Adverse reactions include drowsiness, ataxia, loss of appetite, and slowing of cognition. Renal stones occur in 1% to 2% of patients. The risk of renal stones is greater with a family history. Zonisamide is contraindicated in patients with sulfonamide hypersensitivity.

OTHER ISSUES IN THE MANAGEMENT OF SEIZURES

Education

Treatment includes education of the patient. Emphasize that epilepsy is not a mental illness; it is the condition of having seizures. Discuss driving (guidelines are determined state by state) and avoidance of precipitating factors (e.g., drugs and alcohol, sleep deprivation). Emphasize compliance with medication regimens. Discuss issues of employment and safety, and teach the family simple first-aid tips. Provide educational materials, and refer the patient to the local epilepsy society for information and support. Remember, epilepsy is a chronic condition, and a well-educated patient is a therapeutic ally.

Treatment of the First Seizure

Not all patients with a first seizure require treatment. Overall, about 50% of patients with a first seizure will have a recurrence in the next 3 to 5 years.

Factors that increase the risk of recurrence include:

1. Structural brain lesions.
2. EEG with a definite epileptiform pattern.
3. A history of a prior brain insult.
4. Status epilepticus as a first seizure.

Such patients are usually treated. Patients with a seizure in the setting of drug or alcohol withdrawal, with an acute illness, immediately after a concussion, or with excessive sleep deprivation usually do not need treatment. Patients with two or three unprecipitated seizures have a high risk of recurrence, and should be treated. Patients without structural lesions, with a normal EEG, and with a normal neurologic examination usually do not need treatment after a first seizure.

Discontinuing Antiepileptic Drugs in Seizure-Free Patients

Guidelines by the American Academy of Neurology suggest that patients who are seizure free for 2 to 5 years, with a single type of partial or generalized seizure, normal neurologic examination and IQ, and a normalized EEG, have the greatest chance for successful drug withdrawal. Such patients have a 60% to 70% chance of successful withdrawal. The risks of drug withdrawal should be discussed with the patient, and driving should be restricted during the first few months after tapering off the medication.

Seizures and Pregnancy

The care of the pregnant patient with epilepsy should be undertaken by physicians experienced in this area. Prenatal folate vitamins will decrease the risk of teratogenesis (the dose is at least 1 mg/day). This may be necessary within the first month of pregnancy, usually before a woman is aware she is pregnant. In general, patients taking antiepileptic drugs (AEDs) have a slightly increased risk of complications of pregnancy and minor and major teratogenic defects of the fetus.

Carbamazepine and valproic acid cause an increased risk of neural tube defects, but it is unclear whether higher doses of folate (e.g., 5 mg/day) will reduce this risk. In general, the best AED to be used in a pregnant patient with epilepsy is that drug most likely to best control the seizures. Many AEDs have altered pharmacokinetics in pregnancy, and need careful monitoring. For example, lamotrigine levels may fall dramatically during pregnancy, requiring significant drug adjustments.

Withdrawing medication before pregnancy should be done only in patients considered likely to remain seizure free; withdrawing medication after conception and pregnancy are established adds the risk of seizure to the risk of teratogenesis. Trying to reduce to a single medication before conception is reasonable. Certain AEDs make the risk of neonatal hemorrhage greater, and may be prevented by vitamin K administered to the mother during the last month of pregnancy and to the newborn. Approximately 90% to 95% of children born to mothers with epilepsy are normal.

Seizure Surgery

Surgery is being used more commonly for the treatment of medically intractable epilepsy by the excision of epileptogenic cortex. This therapeutic option usually is considered, when after 1 to 2 years of medication trials do not control seizures, and in cases in which a seizure focus is accessible for surgical treatment. Vagal nerve stimulators and other novel stimulators are also possible treatments for refractory epilepsy.

SOME SPECIFIC SEIZURE SYNDROMES

1. Absence seizures: In childhood, brief (seconds) spells of staring, blinking, tending not to fall, resumption of normal awake state afterwards, EEG 3 per second spike, and wave pattern is typical.
2. Benign occipital epilepsy of childhood (BOEC): Childhood syndrome in young children with prominent headaches, visual aura, and occasional tonic-clonic seizures. EEG shows focal spikes in the occipital regions. Tends to be benign, and children grow out of this syndrome.
3. Juvenile myoclonic epilepsy: An autosomal dominant syndrome, onset in teen years with tonic-clonic seizures (usually in AM), myoclonic seizures, and occasional atypical absence, with 4- to 5-Hz spike and wave on EEG. Responds to valproic acid. Patients do well, but do not grow out of these seizures.
4. Lennox–Gastaut syndrome: Seizures occur in children, usually with cognitive deficits. Seizures are of various types including tonic, atonic, myoclonic, generalized, absence. Seizures are usually difficult to treat.

5. Panayiotopoulos syndrome: A recently better defined child-hood syndrome. It has prominent autonomic features (nausea, vomiting, and syncope) with occasional seizures, occipital spikes, and a benign course. May have autonomic status epilep-ticus, which is difficult to recognize without EEG recording.
6. Rolandic epilepsy: Childhood syndrome with focal seizures, usually at night. May have speech arrest, focal facial twitching, and tonic-clonic seizures. EEG shows focal spikes over the motor cortex. Relatively benign developmental syndrome.
7. Spike wave stupor of the elderly: A syndrome in previously well patients with sudden confusion or fluctuating conscious-ness and EEG continuous spike wave activity. Responds to usual treatment for status epilepticus.
8. West syndrome (hypsarrhythmia): A syndrome in infants and very young children. It is indicated by multiple infantile spasms, very abnormal EEG with high-amplitude waves and multifocal spikes, and is often difficult to treat.

Suggested Readings

Bergin AM, Connolly M. New antiepileptic drug therapies. *Neurol Clin.* 2002;20:1163–1182.

Blume WT. Diagnosis and management of epilepsy. *CMAJ.* 2003;168:441–448.

Dichter M, Buchhalter J. The genetic epilepsies. In: Rosenberg R, Prusiner S, DiMauro S, eds. *The Molecular and Genetic Basis of Neurological and Psychiatric Diseases.* Boston: Butterworth; 2003.

Ferrie CD, Caraballo R, Covanis A, et al. Autonomic status epilepticus in Panayiotopoulos syndrome and other childhood and adult epilepsies: a consensus view. *Epilepsia.* 2007;48:1165–1172.

Glauser T, Ben-Menachem E, Bourgeois B, et al. ILAE treatment guidelines: evidence-based analysis of antiepileptic drug effi-cacy and effectiveness as initial monotherapy for epileptic seizures and syndromes. *Epilepsia.* 2006;47:1094–1120.

Langan Y. Sudden unexpected death in epilepsy (SUDEP): risk factors and case control studies. *Seizure.* 2000;9:179–183.

Meierkord H, Boon P, Engelsen B, et al. EFNS guideline on the management of status epilepticus. *Eur J Neurol.* 2006;13:445–450.

Meierkord H, Holtkamp M. Non-convulsive status epilepticus in adults: clinical forms and treatment. *Lancet Neurol.* 2007;6:329–339.

Sheth RD, Stafstrom CE. Intractable pediatric epilepsy: vagal nerve stimulation and the ketogenic diet. *Neurol Clin.* 2002;20: 1183–1194.

Wiebe S, Blume WT, Girvin JP, et al. A randomized controlled trial of surgery for temporal-lobe epilepsy. *N Engl J Med.* 2001;345: 311–318.

Yerby MS. Clinical care of pregnant women with epilepsy: neural tube defects and folic acid supplementation. *Epilepsia.* 2003; 44(suppl 3):33–40.

Multiple Sclerosis and Related Disorders

CASE

A 34-year-old woman experiences a sudden loss of vision in the left eye that lasts for 2 months, with spontaneous resolution. Three years later, she notices numbness ascending to the waistline that partially resolves after 6 weeks. She is treated with intravenous (IV) methylprednisolone, and improves. Her magnetic resonance imaging (MRI) scan shows periventricular lesions, and her cerebrospinal fluid (CSF) shows oligoclonal bands.

Diagnosis

Relapsing, remitting multiple sclerosis (MS).

Multiple sclerosis (MS) is a relapsing and sometimes progressive disorder that affects primarily the white matter of the central nervous system (CNS—brain and spinal cord). It is an inflammatory disease in which lymphocytes and macrophages damage the myelin sheath, and also may cause axonal damage. It is more common in women, and usually begins between ages 20 and 40 years, although it sometime starts outside this range. MS generally is considered a cell-mediated autoimmune disease directed against myelin components, triggered in some fashion, possibly by an infection. Despite many attempts, an infectious agent has not been identified in MS, and it is not considered an infectious disease.

MAJOR CATEGORIES IN THE CLASSIFICATION OF MULTIPLE SCLEROSIS

1. The relapsing-remitting type, in which patients have discrete attacks of new or worsened neurologic symptoms that come on over a few days. These may resolve over a 4- to 8-week period, with or without corticosteroid treatment. Patients in this category often return to their preattack baseline, but may have residual disability after an attack. They may transition to

secondary progressive disease after some years of disease activity.

Attack = exacerbation = relapse = bout.

Note: An attack of MS is defined as a worsening of neurologic symptoms and or signs over days, not due to infection or increased temperature.

2. The secondary progressive type, in which the patients initially have relapsing-remitting disease, but after some years now have gradual worsening in between discrete attacks. They may have continued attacks, or stop having attacks.

3. The primary progressive type, where the patients are often older at onset, and have a progressive course from onset, without attacks. They tend to have fewer MRI lesions than relapsing-remitting or secondary progressive patients.

Rarer Categories of Multiple Sclerosis

1. The progressive relapsing type, where the patients have gradual neurologic deterioration from the onset, with subsequent superimposed exacerbations.

2. The fulminant type, in which patients have a rapid severe progression, with relapses over a period of months.

SIGNS AND SYMPTOMS

Signs and symptoms occur in multiple anatomic areas of brain and spinal cord affected by the disease.

Common symptoms include the following:

- Sensory (numbness, tingling, heaviness in an extremity, sensory level).
- Visual (visual loss, color vision change, field defects).
- Brainstem (diplopia, dizziness, difficulty swallowing or speaking).
- Motor (weakness, spasticity, cramping, ataxia).
- Bowel and bladder dysfunction.
- Cognitive complaints (fatigue, poor attention, altered memory).

Common signs include the following:

- Corticospinal tract (weakness, spasticity, hyperreflexia, upgoing toes).
- Sensory (vibration loss, decreased pin sense, sensory level).
- Brainstem (nystagmus, internuclear ophthalmoplegia, facial weakness).

- Optic nerve (loss of visual acuity, central scotomas, loss of color vision, optic nerve atrophy, afferent pupillary defect).
- Tremor.

Note: Heat may worsen the symptoms by altering axonal conduction. Transient episodes of neurologic dysfunction (tonic spasms) may occur and last seconds or minutes (transient neurologic events).

DIAGNOSIS

The diagnosis of MS is based primarily on clinical findings reflecting involvement of multiple sites in the brain or spinal cord occurring at different times (i.e., "multiple lesions in time and space"), and an abnormal MRI scan. MRI is the most important laboratory test, and often shows multiple areas of white matter change in the periventricular white matter, corpus callosum, brainstem, and spinal cord. Active MS lesions enhance with gadolinium. Cerebrospinal fluid (CSF) may indicate an inflammatory process with mild pleocytosis and mild protein alteration, increased IgG/albumin ratio and IgG synthesis index, and oligoclonal banding. Evoked potentials (especially those that are visually evoked) are often abnormal, and reflect areas of white matter demyelination. Recently the diagnostic criteria for MS have been modified. In addition to the "two attacks, two clinical findings" criterion, MS also can be diagnosed in patients who have one attack, or progressive disease from the onset. The McDonald criteria allows the diagnosis of MS with a single clinical attack if there are new lesions on subsequent MRI scans.

Based on an MRI, it is now clear that subclinical MS activity occurs when patients appear to be "in remission." New lesions occur on an MRI 5 to10 times as often as there are clinical attacks. Although imperfect, an active MRI and increasing T2 lesion level correlate with attacks and disability. The MRI has a part in clinical decision making, by showing subclinical disease activity. Although MRI lesions can be characteristic of MS, they do not make the diagnosis, and other diseases may cause white matter changes.

DIFFERENTIAL DIAGNOSIS

White matter lesions may be seen in a variety of disorders other than MS.

1. Acute demyelinating encephalomyelitis. A monophasic demyelinating illness may develop after immunizations or viral illnesses. This is usually of rapid onset with severe symptoms, fever, and confusion. Treatment is with high-dose steroids, and sometimes plasmapheresis.

2. Devic disease (neuromyelitis optica). A demyelinating disorder with vasculitic changes in affected areas. Clinically, patients usually have a combination of bilateral optic neuritis and spinal cord involvement sparing brain involvement, but the clinical presentation varies. Attacks of optic neuritis and myelitis may be severe. Cerebrospinal fluid may show a prominent pleocytosis, and increased polymorphonuclear cells. An MRI may show long contiguously extensive lesions over multiple vertebral segments. Recently, a blood test (NMO-IgG) has been shown to be positive in many patients with this clinical picture. Devic disease may require immunosuppressant therapy.

3. Transverse myelitis. A rare and severe condition sometimes after prior infection with spinal cord dysfunction, occurring over hours to days, that is often complete. CSF shows a pleocytosis, but tends to not show oligoclonal banding. The MRI shows longitudinal multisegmental change in the cord. Patients may or may not respond to IV steroids or plasmapheresis. This tends to be a monophasic illness, but some of these patients have relapsing disease, either MS or Devic disease.

4. Vasculitis. Patients with vasculitis-related disorders such as meningovascular syphilis, Sjögren syndrome, lupus erythematosus, Behçet disease, Wegener granulomatosis, and isolated CNS vasculitis may present with an MS-like picture. Asking about the features of the systemic disease, and watching for atypical MRI or clinical appearance, are helpful in diagnosis.

5. Lyme disease. Rarely, infections of the central nervous system may present like MS, but usually have a different CSF and clinical picture. For example, in Lyme disease the typical skin rash, a meningitis presentation, or the presentation of radiculopathy would discriminate it from MS.

6. Structural lesions. Structural lesions such as cervical spondylosis, spinal cord tumor, or posterior fossa tumor may mimic MS. These abnormalities are identified by imaging the affected part of the nervous system.

7. Vitamin B_{12} deficiency. B_{12} deficiency may cause white matter disease and spinal cord disease, but usually as a monophasic illness or progressive illness.

8. Dysmyelinating diseases and CADASIL (cerebral autosomal dominant arteriopathy with subcortical infarcts and leukoencephalopathy).

TREATMENT

Treatment of MS involves two components: (i) disease-modifying therapy directed at the immune system and (ii) symptomatic therapy directed at improving nervous system function (e.g., spasticity).

Disease-Modifying Therapy

Several treatments have been shown to affect the course of the disease and are available to the physician. A hierarchy of therapies is given, depending on the stage and severity of the illness. Most disease-modifying therapies decrease interferon gamma (IFN-g) secretion. Some also induce the secretion of anti-inflammatory cytokines, such as interleukin-4 (IL-4), IL-10, and transforming growth factor beta (TGF-b). Drugs also may affect trafficking or migration of cells into the central nervous system.

1. Acute attacks, if mild, may not require treatment. If they affect function in a significant way, they may be treated with a short course of IV corticosteroids. The most commonly used regimen is a 3- to 7-day course (1,000 mg/day) of IV methylprednisolone given with or without a prednisone taper.
2. Relapsing-remitting disease. Three forms of recombinant interferon beta (beta-1a and 1b) and glatiramer acetate are approved for the treatment of relapsing-remitting MS. They reduce relapses and MRI activity in this group of patients (level 1a evidence). Interferon beta-1b is given subcutaneously as every other day injections. Interferon b-1a is given as three weekly subcutaneous injections, or as a weekly intramuscular injection, and glatiramer acetate is given as a daily subcutaneous injection. Side effects of interferon therapy include injection site reactions, influenza-like symptoms, and worsening of preexisting depression. The choice between the different interferon preparations depends on the patient and individual physician. The most common side effects of glatiramer acetate are mild injection site reactions and in some patients unexplained reactions involving episodes of flushing, chest tightness, shortness of breath, and palpitations. The choice of beginning a relapsing-remitting patient with interferon b versus glatiramer acetate has not been resolved. There is some evidence that higher doses of interferon may be more efficacious. It is recommended that all patients with active relapsing-remitting MS be placed on some form of immunomodulatory therapy.

3. Patients with relapsing-remitting disease who are nonresponders to interferon or glatiramer acetate may be treated with the other medication ("rescue therapy"), depending on how active the disease has become. Those who do not respond include those with continued attacks, increasing disability, and new disease activity on MRI.

   Drugs used as "rescue" therapy include IV pulse methylprednisolone, and immunosuppressant drugs such as pulse cyclophosphamide and mitoxantrone.

   Natalizumab is a monoclonal antibody that blocks lymphocyte entry to the central nervous system. Monthly infusions of this medication have been shown to significantly reduce the attack rate, progression of disability, and MRI activity (level 1a evidence). Risks include occasional anaphylactic reactions and the potential for opportunistic infections such as progressive multifocal leukoencephalopathy. In general, the use of this group of agents should be restricted to clinicians who are experts in the management of MS.

4. Progressive MS. Treatment directed at the progressive phase of MS is more difficult because the disease tends to become worse once the progressive stage has been initiated. Interferon-beta 1b has been shown to have an effect on patients with secondary progressive MS who continue to have attacks (level 1b evidence). Other drugs in use include cyclophosphamide, mitoxantrone methotrexate, and rituximab, depending on the type of progressive disease and how long the patient has been progressive. It has become increasingly recognized that a neurodegenerative component exists in MS, especially in later progressive stages, and immunomodulatory and immunosuppressive therapy may not be effective for this phase of the illness.

Other Treatment Notes

1. Optic neuritis. This may occur during the course of MS, or may be one of the initial symptoms. A recent trial of optic neuritis demonstrated that patients treated with oral prednisone alone were more likely to suffer recurrent episodes of optic neuritis as compared to those treated with methylprednisolone followed by oral prednisone.

   IV methylprednisolone significantly shortened time to recovery of visual function with optic neuritis. These results now make IV methylprednisolone the primary treatment used for optic neuritis. Anaphylactoid reactions and arrhythmias also may occur with methylprednisolone.

2. Fulminating disability. An open study of plasmapheresis in acute episodes of fulminant, central nervous system, inflammatory demyelination showed marked improvement in patients who did not benefit from a course of high-dose IV methylprednisolone, and appears to be an important therapeutic option for this rare subset of patients.

3. Primary progressive MS. This form of MS is difficult to treat and may represent a different pathologic process. There are no randomized trial data to support any particular treatment for this type of MS.

4. Pregnancy. Attacks of MS usually are decreased in frequency during pregnancy, but are increased slightly in the postpartum period. There is no evidence that epidural anesthesia, caesarian section, or normal vaginal birth alter the course of MS. Women should stop disease-modifying therapy 3 months prior to conception, and restart after breast-feeding. Steroids can be used during pregnancy for an attack if necessary.

Symptomatic Therapy

1. Spasticity. Lioresal and tizanidine are effective anti-spastic agents in MS. Regular exercise and stretching are useful. For selected patients, an intrathecal pump of lioresal is effective with a low side effect profile.

2. Pain. Neuropathic pain is relatively common in MS. Treatment is individualized, and depends on the quality of pain, severity, and location. Some medications that may be useful include amitriptyline, nortriptyline, carbamazepine, gabapentin, and pregabalin. Nonsteroidal medication may be tried. Narcotic analgesics are occasionally necessary.

3. Fatigue. Frequent naps and energy conservation are helpful in MS-related fatigue. Make sure there are no nighttime sleep disorders complicating the course. Amantidine and modafinil have been shown to help fatigue in MS. Other agents that are used include methylphenidate (Ritalin) and other stimulant medications in selected patients. A recent randomized trial showed that two aspirin (325 mg) twice a day were effective in reducing MS-related fatigue (level 1b evidence).

4. Transient neurologic events. These events usually last 1 to 2 minutes, and occur several times per day. The patient may confuse them with MS attacks. They consist of paresthesiae or pain in the face or a limb, followed by painful tonic contraction. Another paroxysmal symptom consists of dysarthria and ataxia; usually unilateral limb ataxia, although gait also may be

affected. Paroxysmal phenomena typically subside after a period of weeks. They likely are caused by ephaptic transmission of nerve impulses at sites of previous or new disease activity. Low doses of carbamazepine, phenytoin, or baclofen are usually effective and can be tapered after several weeks.

5. Tremor. Drug therapy has been disappointing. Agents that have been tried include clonazepam, primidone, levetiracetam, topiramate, and propranolol, among many others. Weighted bracelets are often the most practical approach. Surgical thalamotomy has been tried in some cases, with reduction in tremor but often without significant long-term functional improvement.

6. Bladder and bowel dysfunction. Common symptoms include urgency, nocturia, and incontinence; sometimes hesitancy and inability to void occur. One cannot predict the mechanism of bladder dysfunction based on symptoms alone. Thus patients with troublesome bladder symptoms should be referred to a urologist for urodynamic testing. Monitoring for, and treating, urinary tract infections is important. Acidification of the urine with ascorbic acid (vitamin C) or cranberry pills may protect against infections. Chronic antibiotic therapy may lead to resistant organisms. Patients may require intermittent self-catheterization to ensure complete bladder emptying. Indwelling catheterization carries the risk of increased infection. Surgical procedures are sometimes necessary. Constipation is not uncommon in MS, especially in more severely affected, wheelchair-confined patients. Bowel urgency and incontinence are less common. Most patients benefit from increased fluid and roughage in their diet. Metamucil or glycerin suppositories are often helpful. Cathartics should be used only as a last resort.

Suggested Readings

Frohman E, Phillips T, Kokel K, et al. Disease-modifying therapy in multiple sclerosis: strategies for optimizing management. *Neurology*. 2002;8:227–236.

Karussis D, Biermann LD, Bohlega S, et al. A recommended treatment algorithm in relapsing multiple sclerosis: report of an international consensus meeting. *Eur J Neurol*. 2006;13:61–71.

Polman, CH, Reingold SC, Edan G, et al. Diagnostic criteria for multiple sclerosis: 2005 revisions to the "McDonald criteria." *Ann Neurol*. 2005;58:840–846.

Weiner HL. A 21 point hypothesis on the etiology and treatment of multiple sclerosis. *Can J Neurol Sci*.1998;25:93–101.

Weiner HL. Multiple sclerosis is an inflammatory T-cell–mediated autoimmune disease. *Arch Neurol.* 2004;61:1613–1615.

Weiner HL, Cohen JA. Treatment of multiple sclerosis with cyclophosphamide: critical review of clinical and immunologic effects. *Mult Scler.* 2002;8:142–154.

Wingerchuk DM, Lennon VA, Pittock SJ, et al. Revised diagnostic criteria for neuromyelitis optica. *Neurology.* 2006;66: 1485–1489.

Neurology of Diabetes

CASE

A 58-year-old man comes to you because he has "burning" on the skin of his abdomen. His wife says his "belly sticks out on one side." He has diet-controlled diabetes mellitus. He has had an extensive GI workup without any findings. His exam shows absence of superficial abdominal reflexes, with patches of sensory loss over the abdomen and thorax.

Diagnosis

Diabetic thoraco-abdominal polyradiculopathy.

Patients with diabetes frequently have neurologic symptoms. "Neuropathy" is a classic diabetic complication. Most of the neurologic complications of diabetes involve the peripheral nervous system. Cerebrovascular disease and metabolic encephalopathies caused by hypoglycemia or hyperglycemia are the most common central nervous system complications of diabetes.

DIABETIC NEUROPATHY

Distal Polyneuropathy

Distal polyneuropathy is the most common diabetic neuropathy. It presents as a slowly progressive, symmetric, distal ("glove and stocking"), predominantly sensory polyneuropathy. It is caused primarily by metabolic changes in the nerve due to chronically elevated blood sugars. Ankle jerks are generally absent, and vibration sense is diminished; pin and temperature may be decreased distally in the legs more than the arms. The loss of sensation can lead to trophic changes and injury.

Mononeuropathy

Mononeuropathy is a dramatic diabetic neuropathy that probably results from nerve infarction. The onset of motor and sensory loss in one nerve is abrupt, and often painful. The involved nerve may be tender. Prognosis is good, and recovery usually occurs in 4 to 6 months. Treatment is with physical therapy and appropriate support (splints where needed). There is a predilection for certain nerves. The most commonly affected are as follows:

1. *Oculomotor (III) nerve.* The patient has diplopia, and may have pain over the eye. There is an almost total ophthalmoplegia. (Lateral eye movement is spared.) The pupillary fibers are on the outer perimeter of the nerve, and vascular infarction occurs centrally. Thus, the pupil is of normal size and reacts to light (a pupil-sparing third-nerve palsy). *A clue to a "diabetic third" is that the pupillary fibers are often spared.*
2. *Abducens (VI) nerve.* There is an isolated inability to move the eye laterally. Remember, a sixth-nerve palsy may also be the first sign of increased intracranial pressure. (Check for headache and papilledema.)
3. *Femoral nerve.* There is pain in the lateral and anterior thigh, weakness and atrophy of quadriceps (extension at knee), plus weakness of iliopsoas (flexion of hip), and a diminished or absent knee jerk (see Chapter 10).
4. *Radial nerve and peroneal nerve.* There is wristdrop or footdrop, respectively (see Chapter 10).
5. *Facial (VII) nerve.* Bell palsy is more common in diabetics (see Chapter 10).

Entrapment Neuropathy

Entrapment neuropathies such as median nerve at the wrist and ulnar nerve at the elbow are more common in patients with diabetes. Carpal tunnel release may be helpful even in the presence of diabetic neuropathy.

Radiculopathy

Radiculopathy is secondary to involvement of the posterior root outside the spinal cord before it becomes a mixed nerve. Clinically, the patient complains of shooting pains, often confined to a single dermatome. This neuropathy may be difficult to distinguish from disc disease and fortunately resolves spontaneously.

Thoraco-Abdominal Radiculopathy

An important and clinically underappreciated neuropathy is diabetic *thoraco-abdominal radiculopathy*. In this condition, multiple nerve roots are affected, causing a "sunburn" sensation over the abdomen or chest, commonly with focal bulging of the abdominal wall due to associated muscle weakness. It may present early in diabetes, and often is followed by an extensive gastrointestinal and surgical workup before the correct diagnosis is made. Careful sensory and reflex examination shows patchy sensory loss over the abdomen and chest, absent superficial abdominal reflexes, and a lax abdominal musculature. This neuropathy usually improves over several months with control of the diabetes.

Lumbar Plexopathy

Lumbar plexopathy generally is seen in older patients, and consists of pain in the thighs and proximal muscle weakness and wasting; often of sudden onset.

Notable features include increased pain at night and significant weight loss accompanying the onset. Quadriceps and hamstrings also may be weak, and the patient complains of myalgia and dysesthesias in the thighs. Knee and ankle reflexes are usually absent. There is evidence to indicate a microvascular ischemic process, with proximal motor nerves of the lower extremities being affected preferentially. The prognosis is good, with recovery occurring over 6 to 12 months, particularly with optimum control of the diabetes and improved protein intake.

Autonomic Neuropathy

The most common manifestations of *autonomic neuropathy* are orthostatic hypotension (treat with elastic stockings, mineralocorticoids, midodrine, etc.), nocturnal diarrhea, impotence, urinary retention, and abdominal distension. Autonomic neuropathy explains various late problems in diabetes including silent myocardial infarction, loss of "autonomic" symptoms of hypoglycemia, and small, poorly reactive pupils to light with preserved accommodation. Early satiety ("filling up" with small amounts of food), gustatory sweating (profuse sweating only in the face and upper body after a meal), nocturnal diarrhea, and loss of distal limb sweating are other common manifestations of this entity.

COMMENTS ABOUT DIABETES AND THE NERVOUS SYSTEM

1. The physician should make sure that the neuropathies are associated with diabetes, and do not represent symptoms caused by other treatable processes.
2. There is evidence that neuropathies may be prevented or ameliorated by careful blood sugar control in the patient with diabetes, and that insulin is often more effective than oral agents.
3. Based on independent summaries of meta-analyses and randomized trials, medications that were shown to be more effective than placebo for reducing pain in diabetic neuropathy include tricyclic antidepressants, anticonvulsants, topical capsaicin, and lidocaine patches (small case series) (level 1 evidence). Venlafaxine, duloxetine, and pregabalin have also been shown to be useful in diabetic neuropathy pain.
4. Workup of suspected diabetic neuropathy should include assessing duration and control of diabetes, and checking for foot deformities and skin changes. Electromyogram and nerve conduction studies are often helpful in differential diagnosis.
5. It has been reported that some diabetic neuropathies may be treated with anti-inflammatory medication or autoimmune therapy.
6. The restless leg syndrome is a common early manifestation of diabetic neuropathy, and can be treated on its own merits.

CENTRAL NERVOUS SYSTEM DISORDERS ASSOCIATED WITH DIABETES

1. *Diabetic coma* and *hypoglycemia* are common, particularly in patients with insulin-dependent diabetes. Remember to draw blood to test the blood sugar level, and administer 50% glucose intravenously to all patients presenting with coma of uncertain cause.
2. Patients with hypoglycemia may present with behavioral disturbances, seizures, and focal neurologic deficits that clear after glucose administration. Beware of the "stroke alert" patient who actually has a blood sugar of 30.
3. Treatment of *hyperglycemia* and coma may result in hypokalemia and a flaccid paralysis.
4. Cerebral edema may occur in both diabetic ketoacidosis and in nonketotic hyperglycemic states.

5. Occasionally, patients with diabetes with highly elevated sugars (e.g., hyperosmotic nonketotic states) will have continuous focal motor seizure activity that resists treatment until the glucose is controlled (epilepsia partialis continua).

6. Patients with diabetes are at increased risk for cerebrovascular disease, with both large- and small-vessel atherosclerosis.

Suggested Readings

McCall AL. Diabetes mellitus and the central nervous system. *Int Rev Neurobiol.* 2002;51:415–453.

Watson CP, Moulin D, Watt-Watson J, et al. Controlled-release oxycodone relieves neuropathic pain: a randomized controlled trial in painful diabetic neuropathy. *Pain.* 2003;105:71–78.

Wein TH, Albers JW. Diabetic neuropathies. *Phys Med Rehab Clin North Am.* 2001;12:307–320.

Wong MC, Chung JW, Wong TK. Effects of treatments for symptoms of painful diabetic neuropathy: systematic review. *BMJ.* 2007;335:87.

23 Malignancy and the Nervous System

CASE

A 45–year-old, right-handed swimming coach presents to the emergency room with two generalized tonic-clonic seizures. He is confused, has trouble forming words, and has a mild right pronator drift. His MRI shows an irregularly enhancing mass in the left frontal white matter.

Diagnosis

Probable glioblastoma multiforme; left frontal lobe.

Malignancies may affect the nervous system in a variety of ways. Primary and metastatic tumors may affect the brain, spinal cord, and peripheral nervous system directly. Distant tumors may affect various neurologic systems due to metabolic changes, or due to paraneoplastic effects. Radiation may cause injury to radiosensitive neural structures. Chemotherapies have a variety of effects on nervous system tissues. Patients with malignancies are often at increased risk of stroke. Finally, nutritional disorders in cancer patients can lead to injury to the nervous system.

SIGNS AND SYMPTOMS OF BRAIN TUMOR

These signs and symptoms apply to primary and metastatic central nervous system (CNS) tumors.

1. Does the patient have *headache*? Headache is one of the most common symptoms, present in approximately two thirds of patients. It often occurs in the morning, when intracranial pressure is higher.
2. Other signs and symptoms include seizures, personality changes, hemiplegia, and visual disturbances. Mental changes, especially memory loss and decreased alertness, are often important subtle clues of intracranial tumor.
3. Patients may have a *gait disturbance*.

4. Seizures associated with tumor are characteristically focal. They may be "Jacksonian"—a focal seizure that begins in one extremity, then "marches" along one side of the body. It may become a generalized convulsion. **New-onset seizures in a middle-aged adult are often caused by a brain tumor.**
5. Check for *papilledema*, or sixth-nerve paresis caused by increased intracranial pressure.
6. Sometimes there may be bleeding within a tumor or vessel occlusion, creating the clinical picture of a stroke. Some tumors have a propensity to bleed (e.g., melanoma, hypernephroma, and choriocarcinoma).

PRIMARY BRAIN TUMORS

Primary brain tumors, although uncommon, are a significant cause of death in middle-aged adults. The most common types are glioblastoma multiforme, astrocytoma, meningioma, and pituitary adenoma. Primary central nervous system (CNS) lymphoma is becoming more common, particularly in patients with acquired immune deficiency syndrome (AIDS).

Glioblastoma Multiforme (GBM)

Glioblastoma multiforme comprises 20% of all intracranial tumors. It is usually located in the hemispheres in adults, with peak incidence in middle age. It may present with headache, seizure, or a personality change. It is a neoplasm of astrocytic-type cells, and is a vascular tumor with irregular enhancement on MRI and computed tomography (CT). Irrespective of treatment, it carries a poor prognosis for long-term survival.

Astrocytoma

Astrocytoma is a slower-growing astrocytic tumor with a better long-term prognosis than GMB, but cure is rare. Astrocytoma may form large cysts. In approximately half of patients, it presents with seizures.

Meningioma

Meningioma is a benign tumor of the dura, located over the surface of the brain (convexity, wing of the sphenoid, skull base), in the spinal canal as an intradural/extramedullary lesion, and rarely in an intra-ventricular location. It is more common in women and in the elderly. Thoracic spinal meningioma occurs particularly in elderly women. Meningiomas enhance on MRI and CT, and angiography shows a tumor blush.

Pituitary Adenoma

Pituitary adenoma is an endocrine tumor that may cause amen-orrhea, acromegaly, Cushing disease, or rarely, hyperthyroidism. It may be nonsecreting, causing symptoms by pressure on the optic chiasm and/or normal pituitary gland. Classically, it causes a bitemporal hemianopsia (loss of temporal fields of vision) because of compression of the nasal retinal fibers passing through the chiasm.

Primary Central Nervous System Lymphoma

Primary CNS lymphoma is a B-cell tumor with a periventricular localization that may involve the eye in 20% of cases. (Vitreous biopsy may be diagnostic.) It is common in patients with AIDS, and occurs in other immunosuppressed patients. It is often deep in the brain and usually multicentric. It is rapidly progressive, and treated by stereotactic biopsy, radiation, steroids, and chemother-apy. It is usually unresectable. In patients infected with the human immunodeficiency virus, it may be difficult to distinguish lym-phoma from toxoplasmosis; stereotactic biopsy may be helpful. Prognosis is poor when AIDS is present. Because steroid therapy may lyse CNS lymphoma, delay use of steroids until after biopsy if CNS lymphoma is suspected.

INTRACRANIAL METASTASES

Which Tumors Invade the Brain?

Up to 25% of patients with cancer have cerebral metastases at autopsy. Metastatic tumor reaches the brain through hematoge-nous spread, and generally after first invading the lung. This accounts for the high incidence of intracranial metastases with *lung* and *breast* tumors. Other tumors that metastasize to brain include melanoma, hypernephroma, and GI malignancies

LABORATORY INVESTIGATION FOR BRAIN TUMOR

1. MRI with gadolinium enhancement is the most sensitive test for detection of brain tumor, especially in the posterior fossa. Contrast-enhanced MRI is particularly useful if leptomeningeal metastases are suspected.
2. Arteriography is rarely necessary for diagnosis. Arteriography may be helpful before surgery on a meningioma to delineate the vascular supply of the tumor.
3. There is increasing use of stereotactic brain biopsy as a method of establishing the correct diagnosis with low morbidity; particularly for lesions that are not considered resectable. However, pathologic diagnosis sometimes may be difficult, because of the small amount of tissue obtained with this kind of biopsy.

TREATMENT OF BRAIN TUMOR

The treatment of *primary brain tumor* depends on the tumor type and location:

1. Meningiomas are usually surgically removable.
2. Low-grade astrocytomas and oligodendrogliomas are best treated by surgery plus irradiation.
3. High-grade astrocytomas (glioblastoma multiforme) are treated by resection plus irradiation or, depending on location, partial removal plus irradiation. There is increasing use of chemotherapy—such as 1, 3-bis-(2 chloroethyl) 1-nitrosouria (BCNU) intravenously, or as Gliadel wafers implanted at the time of resection—which prolongs survival. Adjuvant chemotherapy may be useful in oligodendroglioma and astrocytomas. Chemotherapy trials are available for most patients with primary brain tumor.
4. Tumors showing symptomatic mass effect may be treated with dexamethasone.

Newer radiotherapy techniques have included radioactive implants and stereotactic radiosurgery (linear accelerator or gamma knife).

1. In meningiomas, surgical resection of this tumor is usually curative, unless only partial removal is possible or anaplastic pathology is present. Certain meningiomas that are benign cannot be completely resected because of their location, such as in the cavernous sinus or growing into the sagittal sinus.

2. In pituitary adenomas, treatment is surgical; other treatment modalities include radiotherapy and endocrine replacement therapy. Prolactin secreting tumors may respond to suppression of prolactin release by dopamine agonists.

3. In primary CNS lymphomas, a multidrug-chemotherapy combination, including methotrexate, procarbazine, vincristine, dexamethasone, and cytarabine plus radiation therapy, has been shown to produce an increase in median survival of 41 months. This is compared with 10 months for patients receiving radiotherapy alone. Newer regimens with high-dose methotrexate have also been used.

4. In patients with *metastatic brain tumor*, one must first determine whether the brain is involved by single or multiple metastases. MRI with gadolinium is the most sensitive test. Documented *multiple metastases* are treated with steroids and whole brain irradiation. Symptoms are ameliorated with steroids to reduce cerebral edema. One randomized study showed similar efficacy using dexamethasone 1 mg. q.i.d. and 4 mg. q.i.d., with a reduced side-effect profile in the low-dose regimen. Higher doses are used for impending herniation. Irradiation improves length and quality of survival. Chemotherapy may be added.

Treatment of a *single metastasis* is surgical, if the patient is a good operative candidate and the lesion is surgically accessible. In addition to offering palliation, other disease processes sometimes are found at operation (e.g., subdural hematoma, brain abscess, primary brain tumor). Radiosurgery provides another approach to single metastases less than 3 cm in diameter, and is sometimes used with 2 to 4 metastases.

METASTATIC TUMOR TO THE SPINAL CORD

Management

Metastatic tumor to the cord (generally epidural implant) may compress the cord; it constitutes a neurologic emergency (see Chapter 9).

LEUKEMIA AND LYMPHOMA

Leukemia and lymphoma are malignant processes frequently associated with nervous system dysfunction, and may invade the brain and spinal cord. With more effective treatment and with patients living longer, there has been an increasing incidence of CNS complications.

Leukemia

Leukemia is associated with a triad of neurologic complications:

1. *Intracranial hemorrhage* is common in leukemia, and is usually related to a low platelet count or a high leukocyte count (more than 100,000/mm). Intracranial bleeding occurs in multiple areas (not usually one, as in hypertensive bleeding) and is often associated with systemic bleeding.
2. Leukemic infiltration of the meninges (of brain and spinal cord) and nerve roots is common, and may occur when the patient is in hematologic remission. Meningeal leukemia usually presents as headache, nausea, and vomiting, secondary to increased intracranial pressure (there may be papilledema); seizures, visual disturbances, and ataxia also occur. Cranial nerve palsies occur (commonly III, VI, and VII).

   Diagnosis is made by lumbar puncture (LP). Look for elevated pressure, leukemic cells, elevated protein, and decreased sugar. MRI with gadolinium may detect leukemic infiltration, and is particularly useful in detecting leptomeningeal spread.

   Treatment with intrathecal methotrexate and radiotherapy is usually effective, and may be given prophylactically to patients with leukemia in hematologic remission, before CNS complications occur.
3. *Infection.* These patients are prone to CNS infection; usually bacterial (e.g., *Listeria*) and fungal (e.g., *Cryptococcus*). Whenever CNS symptoms are present, even if they are only drowsiness and headache, perform a lumbar puncture to look for meningeal leukemia or infection; after excluding a mass lesion by CT scan or MRI.

Lymphoma

Patients with *lymphoma* are subject to the same complications as those with leukemia, except for intracerebral hemorrhage. Leptomeningeal spread is common in non-Hodgkin lymphoma.

Spinal cord compression by lymphoma is especially common, as are compressive syndromes in other parts of the nervous system: brachial plexus, recurrent laryngeal nerve (vocal cord paralysis), phrenic nerve, cervical sympathetics (Horner syndrome), and lumbosacral roots.

Treatment of choice is radiation and chemotherapy.

Note: Meningeal involvement by tumors other than lymphoma and leukemia (*carcinomatous meningitis*) occurs most commonly with breast cancer.

NONMETASTATIC COMPLICATIONS OF MALIGNANCY

Paraneoplastic Syndromes

Paraneoplastic syndromes are a unique group of disorders that reflects the remote effects of malignancy on the nervous system. The etiology of these distant effects varies, and may be related to immunologic, hormonal, or toxic factors elaborated by the tumor.

A variety of unique neurologic syndromes may be the first manifestation of a malignancy elsewhere.

Distant neurologic dysfunction as a result of malignancy is known as a paraneoplastic syndrome.

Symptoms associated with these syndromes sometimes disappear when the primary tumor is removed. Certain neoplasms such as small-cell lung cancer are more commonly associated with neurologic findings.

Paraneoplastic Encephalomyelitis (PEM)

This is an immune inflammatory disorder that can affect any part of the CNS, the dorsal root ganglia, and the autonomic nervous system.

Various clinical syndromes can be seen, including:

1. Limbic encephalitis (hippocampal involvement).
2. Cerebellar degeneration (Purkinje cell involvement).
3. Brainstem encephalitis.
4. Sensory neuronopathy (dorsal root ganglion involvement).
5. Autonomic disorder.

Often two or more of these syndromes can occur at the same time. In general, treatment is aimed at eradicating the primary tumor if possible. Anecdotal immunologic treatments have included steroids, plasmapheresis, and IVIG, but there are no randomized trials to objectively guide therapy in these disorders.

Paraneoplastic Cerebellar Degeneration (PCD)

With PCD, there is unsteadiness in gait and difficulty using limbs, progressing to slurred speech and trouble eating. Symptoms usually progress over weeks. PCD is usually seen with tumors of the lung, ovary, and breast.

Although the cerebellar dysfunction is most striking, there may be other evidence of associated CNS dysfunction including mental changes, muscle weakness, peripheral neuropathy, and extensor plantar responses. Anti-Purkinje cell antibodies have been detected in the serum and CSF of some of these patients, and patients with such antibodies have a more rapid course.

Lambert–Eaton Myasthenic Syndrome (LEMS)

LEMS is frequently associated with small cell lung carcinoma in men. It presents as a generalized proximal weakness and easy fatigability. Associated features include dry mouth, impotence, and peripheral paresthesias. Trouble with eye movements or difficulty swallowing is less common.

LEMS is a presynaptic disorder of the neuromuscular junction, whereas myasthenia gravis affects the postsynaptic junction. P/Q type voltage-gated calcium channel antibodies may be present. Limited evidence from randomized trials shows that either 3, 4-diaminopyridine or intravenous immunoglobulin improves muscle strength scores in patients with LEMS. LEMS may occur in the absence of malignancy; this syndrome has an autoimmune basis. Patients with this syndrome may be abnormally sensitive to muscle relaxants used in anesthesia, at times with life-threatening respiratory suppression.

Sensory Neuronopathy

This is a paraneoplastic disorder with degeneration of dorsal root ganglion cells. There is usually numbness and tingling of the upper and lower extremities, associated with a sensory ataxia. Facial numbness may occur early, as this is not a "length-dependent" neuropathy. Reflexes are absent, and there may be proximal muscle wasting in the lower extremities. A sensorimotor neuropathy also has been associated with malignancy.

Opsoclonus-Myoclonus (OM)

Opsoclonus (a peculiar jerking of the eyes to and fro), and myoclonus (a sudden jerking of large muscle groups), may be seen as a remote effects of cancer (neuroblastoma in young children, various tumors in adults).

Limbic Encephalitis

Limbic encephalitis is a rare paraneoplastic syndrome. It usually affects the hippocampus, and presents with short-term memory loss, seizures, confusion, irritability, depression, apathy, and altered sleep. Patients may develop seizures; including nonconvulsive status. CSF is non-specifically abnormal, and MRI may show changes in the hippocampi.

Dermatomyositis

Dermatomyositis is frequently associated with neoplasm, and may antedate the appearance of the tumor. The myositis presents as proximal muscle weakness. The muscles are usually not tender. There is an associated skin rash, with a purplish rash of the eyelids (heliotrope rash), and scaly lesions over the knuckles (erythematous). If tumor eradication is impossible or does not help, steroids may be of benefit.

Paraneoplastic Antibodies

There is now a growing list of antibodies that serve as markers of paraneoplastic syndromes, and that may hint at the presence of malignancy.

The well-characterized paraneoplastic antibodies include:

1. Hu (ANNA1).
2. Yo (PCA1).
3. CV2/CRMP5.
4. Ri (ANNA2).
5. Ma2.
6. Amphiphysin.

Less well-characterized antibodies include Tr, Zic4, PCA2, and ANNA3. These antibodies may provide a clue as to the location and tissue type of occult malignancies causing paraneoplastic syndromes (Table 23.1).

Metabolic Encephalopathy

Patients with cancer are prone to develop lethargy, confusion, and behavior disturbances as the result of metabolic abnormalities related to, but not directly resulting from, the underlying cancer.

■ TABLE 23.1. Paraneoplastic Antibodies

Antibody	Associated Syndrome	Most Frequent Tumor
Hu	PEM, PCD Sensory neuronopathy	Small cell lung cancer (SCLC)
Yo	PCD	Ovary, breast
CV2/CRMP5	Several	SCLC, thymoma
Ri	PCD, OM, brainstem encephalitis	Breast, gynecologic, SCLC
Ma2	PEM	Testicular, SCLC
Amphiphysin	Stiff person syndrome, PEM	Breast, SCLC

Radiologic assessment depends on the tumor type and location. If radiologic assessment is negative, PDG-PET is useful in detecting an occult malignancy.

Examples include: uremia, hepatic and respiratory failure, electrolyte disturbances such as hypercalcemia, hyponatremia, and hypoglycemia, and drug overdoses.

Patients with cancer also are prone to develop infections of various types, and sepsis may cause a metabolic encephalopathy. Metabolic brain disease is suggested by lethargy, clouding of consciousness, a fluctuating picture, myoclonus, a lack of focal signs, and confirmatory laboratory studies such as a normal CT scan or MRI and an abnormal EEG that shows bilateral slowing without focal features.

Vascular Disorders

Patients with cancer are prone to develop vascular disorders, such as cerebral infarction secondary to disseminated intravascular coagulation, venous sinus thromboses, or emboli from nonbacterial endocarditis (marantic endocarditis). They also are prone to intracerebral, subarachnoid, or subdural hemorrhage caused by thrombocytopenia or other coagulation disorder. Sometimes, thrombosis in patients with cancer may not respond to treatment with warfarin and requires subcutaneous heparin.

RADIATION

Radiation can affect nervous system tissue in various ways. The frequency and severity of injury depend on the radiation dose and fractionation, preexisting neurologic injury, and patient characteristics such as age and white matter disease.

Syndromes following brain radiation treatment:

1. Acute encephalopathy: within 2 weeks of starting treatment, vasogenic edema, headache, somnolence, worsening deficit may occur. Steroids rapidly improve the syndrome, which is reversible.
2. Early-delayed encephalopathy: within 1 to 6 months after treatment; new areas of contrast enhancement, surrounding edema. Drowsiness and cognitive impairment occur. This is reversible, and may be improved with steroids.
3. Late-delayed encephalopathy: within months to years after brain radiation. Patients develop progressive mental slowing, poor memory, urinary incontinence, apathy, and occasionally, pyramidal and extrapyramidal disorders. Atrophy and white matter changes are seen in MRI. There is no known therapy for this progressive disorder.
4. Focal radiation necrosis: may occur months to years after focal RT. Histology shows focal white-matter necoris with hyalinized thickening of vessels, and fibrinoid necrosis. There are vascular changes with narrowed lumens, thrombosis, hemorrhages. MRI and CT show a contrast-enhancing lesion with mass effect. May be mistaken for tumor. No current imaging modality can definitively discriminate the two.

PLEXUS LESIONS

Both tumor and radiation can affect the plexus structure. Discriminating radiation injury from tumor is key in planning treatment. There are some clinical and EMG findings that help to discriminate tumor-induced injury from radiation (Table 23.2).

■ TABLE 23.2. Neoplastic Versus Radiation-Induced Plexopathies

Symptom/Sign	Tumor	Radiation
Pain prominent	Common	Uncommon
Lower trunk involved	Common	Uncommon
Horner syndrome present	Common	Uncommon
Mass on MRI	Common	None
Myokymia (EMG)	Uncommon	Common

BONE MARROW TRANSPLANTATION

Bone marrow transplantation (BMT) carries several risks:

1. Toxicity from chemotherapy.
2. Infection caused by immune suppression.
3. Bleeding related to thrombocytopenia.
4. Graft versus host disease.

   More than half the patients undergoing BMT develop neurologic dysfunction. The most common neurologic side effect is a metabolic encephalopathy. Central nervous system (CNS) bacterial, viral, or fungal infection may occur as a result of profound immunosuppression (e.g., cytomegalovirus encephalitis, herpes zoster radiculitis). There may be thrombotic infarction or hemorrhage.

   Other neurologic syndromes such as mononeuritis multiplex, transverse myelitis, and myositis may be related to graft versus host disease. In children, cerebral atrophy, neuropsychologic dysfunction, and leukoencephalopathy also have been reported following BMT.

OTHER COMPLICATIONS

Cancer patients may develop side effects secondary to chemotherapeutic agents (especially vincristine and cisplatinum). Providing a long list of chemotherapies and their neurologic symptoms is not particularly helpful.

When considering chemotherapy-induced neurologic disorders, it is best to review the specific medications used in the patient and check whether they are known to cause such a syndrome.

Suggested Readings

Chang JE, Robins HI, Mehta MP. Therapeutic advances in the treatment of brain metastases. *Clin Adv Hematol Oncol.* 2007;5: 54–64.

Li B, Yu J, Suntharalingam M. Comparison of three treatment options for single brain metastasis from lung cancer. *Int J Cancer.* 2000;90:37–45.

Maddison P, Newsom-Davis J. Treatment for Lambert-Eaton myasthenic syndrome. *Cochrane Database Syst Rev.* 2005;2: CD003279.

Rees J. Neurological manifestations of malignant disease. *Hosp Med.* 2000;61:319–325.

Stupp R, Mason WP, van den Bent MJ, et al. Radiotherapy plus concomitant and adjuvant temozolomide for glioblastoma. *N Engl J Med.* 2005;352:987–996.

Vedeler CA, Antoine JC, Giometto B, et al. Management of paraneoplastic neurological syndromes: report of the EFNS task force. *Eur J Neurol.* 2006;13:682–690.

Central Nervous System Infections

Central nervous system (CNS) infections are suggested by a constellation of signs, symptoms, and laboratory studies. The major groups of CNS infections include:

1. Bacterial meningitis.
2. Viral meningitis.
3. Chronic meningitis.
4. Acute encephalitis.
5. Brain abscess.

See Chapter 25 for the treatment of acquired immune deficiency virus (AIDS)-related CNS infections.

HISTORY

The diagnosis of *meningitis* (inflammation of the meninges) is suggested when history includes fever, headache, and stiff neck.

1. *Acute bacterial meningitis* is a neurologic emergency, with symptoms developing over hours or days. Cerebrospinal fluid (CSF) studies show a neutrophilic pleocytosis, low glucose compared with blood glucose, and high protein. Cultures or bacterial antigens are positive. CSF pressure may be high. **Delay in diagnosis and treatment can lead to permanent injury or death.**
2. *Viral meningitis* is suggested by the constellation of fever, headache, and stiff neck; the cerebrospinal fluid (CSF) features include a lymphocytic pleocytosis, normal sugar, and negative culture for bacteria.
3. *Chronic meningitis* has a more indolent presentation, and may be associated with cranial nerve palsies, cognitive changes, or stroke-like events. The diagnosis of encephalitis (evidence of brain parenchymal involvement) is suggested, when the history includes fever, the acute onset of mental status changes (ranging from confusion to coma), seizures, and focal neurologic signs such as paralysis, acute psychosis, or aphasia. CSF shows

a lymphocytic pleocytosis with normal sugar. PCR for herpes simplex or other viral causes of encephalitis may be positive. MRI may show abnormalities in certain parts of the brain, such as the temporal lobe depending on the type of encephalitis.

4. The diagnosis of *brain abscess* is suggested by subacute fever, headache, focal signs or seizures, and signs of increased intracranial pressures. Fever is seen in approximately 50% of adults and up to 80% of children with brain abscess. Imaging shows a focal ring enhancing mass lesion or multiple lesions. **CSF studies should not be performed to avoid herniation due to mass effect.**

Pursue the Following Points in the History:

1. Has there been a recent respiratory or gastrointestinal infection?
2. Has the patient had a recent infectious illness that may progress to meningitis (e.g., otitis media leading to pneumococcal meningitis)? Has the patient had a positive reaction to purified protein derivative, or known exposure to tuberculosis?
3. Has the patient been exposed to others with infectious illness (e.g., meningococcus or *Haemophilus influenzae*)?
4. Has there been recent travel to another state (e.g., exposure to mosquitoes causing arbovirus-associated encephalitis), or another country (cysticercosis in Central America)?
5. Has there been a subtle personality change and low-grade fever (e.g., in chronic meningitis such as *Cryptococcus*)?
6. What is the patient's occupation (e.g., painter exposed to *Cryptococcus* in pigeon droppings)?
7. Does an *underlying disease* predispose the patient to CNS infection?
   - Lymphoma, leukemia.
   - Other malignancy.
   - Renal failure.
   - HIV/AIDS, other immunodeficiency states.
   - Alcoholism.
   - Diabetes.
   - Post-transplant patient.
   - Asplenic (functional or surgical).

8. Is the patient receiving a drug(s) that predisposes to infection?
   - Chemotherapy.
   - Immunosuppressant or immunomodulator.
   - Corticosteroids.

9. Has the patient had a recent illness such as mumps, or chickenpox that may be followed by meningitis or meningoencephalitis?

10. Is the patient bacteremic, or has the patient recently been bacteremic? This increases the chances of secondary CNS infection.
11. Has there been a recent head injury?
12. Has there been a recent neurosurgical procedure or penetrating skull trauma?
13. Has there been a recent insect bite leading to Lyme disease, or rickettsial infection, which mimics bacterial meningitis?

PHYSICAL AND NEUROLOGIC EXAMINATION

1. Check vital signs. Temperature may be higher in bacterial than in viral CNS infection. Herpes simplex encephalitis often results in a high fever (104°F–105°F). Tachycardia is seen in bacterial and viral CNS infection.
2. Check eardrums; examine sinuses for tenderness.
3. Check for stiff neck. Look for Kernig sign (with thigh flexed on abdomen, patient resists knee extension), or Brudzinski sign (attempt to flex the neck, results in reflex flexion of the knee and hip). Remember that the elderly, infants, and immunosuppressed patients may have meningitis without prominent meningeal signs. Comatose patients may not have meningismus.
4. Look for stigmata of chronic liver disease, and chronic lung disease as a predisposing factor for CNS infection.
5. Look for peripheral signs of embolization in a patient suspected of having subacute bacterial endocarditis or staphylococcal septicemia.
6. Examine the heart carefully (e.g., changing murmur in subacute bacterial endocarditis with valvular disease as source of septic embolism).
7. Examine for lymph-node enlargement or splenomegaly. These signs may suggest a lymphoproliferative disorder, in which CNS infections commonly are seen.
8. Is there evidence of CSF rhinorrhea caused by a defect or fracture in the cribriform plate?
9. Examine for petechial or purpuric lesions caused by meningococcemia, or staphylococcal bacteremia.

LABORATORY

1. All patients suspected of having meningitis should have a lumbar puncture (LP), and treatment with antibiotics as soon as

possible (Table 24.1). Record the opening pressure. If focal neurologic symptoms or signs are present and brain abscess is a consideration, obtain a contrast-enhanced computed tomography (CT) or magnetic resonance imaging (MRI) scan first, but do not allow significant delay when there is a high likelihood of meningitis. If meningitis is a reasonable possibility and imaging is necessary, it may be appropriate to give IV antibiotics immediately. Blood cultures should be drawn before antibiotics are begun. See Chapter 30 for a discussion of CSF examination.

In addition, note the following points regarding meningitis and encephalitis:

- CSF pressure is usually moderately elevated in bacterial meningitis (200 to 300 mm H_2O), and mildly elevated in viral meningitis or encephalitis.
- Cell count in untreated bacterial meningitis may range from 100 to 10,000/mm^3 with a predominance of neutrophils; the fluid is usually cloudy. In viral meningitis, cell counts of 10 to 1,000/mm^3 with a predominance of mononuclear cells are expected.
- CSF glucose is usually less than 40 mg/dL in bacterial or tuberculous meningitis (or less than 60% of simultaneously obtained blood glucose), whereas it is usually normal, or only modestly reduced in viral meningitis or encephalitis.
- CSF protein is usually higher than 100 mg/dL in bacterial meningitis, whereas a mild elevation (50–100 mg/dL) is expected in viral meningitis or encephalitis. A mild elevation also may be encountered in partially treated meningitis.
- Elevated CSF lactate levels are commonly encountered in patients with meningitis following neurosurgical procedures.

■ TABLE 24.1. Differential of Major Meningitis Syndromes

	Bacterial Meningitis	Viral Meningitis	Fungal, TB
Pressure	Increased	Normal	Increased
Cell count	Thousands, PMN	< 500, usually lymphocytes	Hundreds, mononuclear cells
Micro	Gram stain often positive	No organisms	India ink 80% effective for fungi; AFB 40% for TB
Glucose	Decreased	Normal	Decreased
Protein	Increased + +	Slight increase	May be + + + increased

- Gram stain usually detects the causative organism in bacterial meningitis. India ink stain is helpful in diagnosing cryptococcal meningitis, as are CSF and serum cryptococcal antigens. Bacterial antigens can be detected in the spinal fluid by a variety of special techniques and may be helpful if the patient received antibiotic therapy before the LP.

2. Routine laboratory tests may offer clues. The white blood cell count is usually markedly elevated in bacterial meningitis and mildly elevated or normal in viral meningitis.

3. Check for hyponatremia, caused by inappropriate antidiuretic hormone secretion, as a complicating feature in a meningitis patient with increasing lethargy.

4. Chest radiograph may demonstrate a source of CNS infection (e.g., pneumonia or bronchiectasis).

5. The electroencephalogram (EEG) may be normal or slightly slow in meningitis and encephalitis, but it often shows focal features in brain abscess and paroxysmal features in the temporal lobe in herpes simplex encephalitis.

6. CT and MRI scans are usually normal in uncomplicated meningitis, but are often focally abnormal in herpes simplex encephalitis (temporal lobe). They may demonstrate complications of meningitis such as subdural fluid collections, hydrocephalus, or cerebral infarction.

7. In patients with suspected viral CNS infections, obtain a serum specimen acutely, and save to compare with convalescent sera for an increase in antibody titers (e.g., in mumps infection).

8. In suspected enterovirus CNS infection (Coxsackie, Echo), the virus often is detected in stool specimens. Mumps virus may be isolated from saliva, throat washings, or CSF.

9. Bacteremia is present in many patients with bacterial meningitis and should be detected by appropriate blood cultures.

10. Beware of coagulopathy in patients with fulminant meningitis (especially meningococcus).

11. Use PCR (polymerase chain reaction) to identify herpes simplex.

TREATMENT

Bacterial Meningitis

The mainstay of treatment of bacterial meningitis is intravenous antibiotics (Table 24.2). For suspected undiagnosed bacterial meningitis in adults, start ceftriaxone 2 g intravenously (IV) every

■ **TABLE 24.2. Antibiotics Used for Meningitis**

Organism	Appropriate Antibiotics
Streptococcus pneumoniae	Vancomycin + 3rd-gen. cephalosporin
Strep. Agalactiae	Ampicillin or pen G, or 3rd-gen. cephalosporin
Neisseria meningitidis	3rd-gen. cephalosporin or pen G, ampicillin
Haemophilus influenzae	3rd-gen. cephalosporin or chloramphenicol
Staphylococcus aureus	Nafcillin ± rifampin or vancomycin
Listeria monocytogenes	Ampicillin, trimethoprim-sulfamethoxazole
Escherichia coli, Klebsiella	3rd-gen. cephalosporin or meropenem
Proteus	Ceftriaxone, meropenem
Pseudomonas	Ceftazidime and aminoglycoside, meropenem

Grade A recommendations (Tunkel, 2004). The final selection of antimicrobial medications should be based on careful review of microbiology results, patient drug allergies, and renal status.
From Tunkel AR, Hartman BJ, Kaplan SL, et al. Practice guidelines for the management of bacterial meningitis. *Clin Infect Dis.* 2004;39:1267–1284.

12 hours. If penicillin-resistant pneumococcus is a concern, vancomycin 1 g IV every 12 hours should be administered, until susceptibilities are available.

If *Listeria* is a consideration (immunosuppressed individual), ampicillin 2 g IV, every 4 hours should be added to the regimen. Appropriate dosing modifications for age and renal function need to be considered for all patients. For those with a severe allergy to beta-lactam antibiotics, chloramphenicol may be prescribed. Remember, if a lumbar puncture is delayed for any reason, consider giving empiric antibiotics before LP.

Early treatment is crucial in these patients.

Other measures include the following:

1. Seizures are common in meningitis, and usually are treated with intravenous phenytoin or fos-phenytoin.
2. Fluid restriction to 1,200 to 1,500 mL/day may be needed to reduce brain swelling, or to control the syndrome of inappropriate antidiuretic hormone.
3. Early use of dexamethasone 0.15 mg/kg IV every 6 hours for 2 days in children, and dexamethasone 10 mg IV q6h for 4 days in adults, may reduce unfavorable outcomes in adults and children with bacterial meningitis.
4. Standard infection-control precautions (gloves, hand-washing, face/eye/mouth shield) and additional droplet precautions are essential for all cases of known or suspected meningitis.

5. Family members, medical personnel, and others with close contact to patients with meningococcal meningitis should receive prophylaxis with one of the following regimens:
   • Ciprofloxacin 500-mg single oral dose (adults only).
   • Rifampin 600 mg orally every 12 hours for 2 days.
   • Ceftriaxone 250 mg intramuscularly (adult dosing; check for appropriate pediatric dosing).

Viral Meningitis/Encephalitis

1. Treatment of *viral meningitis* is supportive.
2. In cases of nonherpetic *viral encephalitis*, treatment is also supportive, and directed at possible complications. For herpes simplex encephalitis, acyclovir has greatly improved morbidity and mortality. Usual dosage is 10 mg/kg every 8 hours IV, with vigorous hydration to avoid nephrotoxicity.
3. Take meticulous care to promptly and completely dispose of needles and syringes, and precautions should be undertaken in handling stool specimens in those with enteroviral infection.
4. Isolate patients suspected of having measles, chickenpox, or rubella.
5. Treat fever with acetaminophen or aspirin. A cooling blanket may be helpful for extreme hyperthermia.
6. Treat seizures that accompany encephalitis.
7. The first cases of West Nile encephalitis in North America were reported in the summer of 1999. Since that time, the disease has become endemic in this area. West Nile virus is a member of the flavivirus family. Transmission to humans occurs following the bite of infected mosquitoes and, in rare cases, following blood transfusion or organ transplantation from an infected source patient. Most infections are asymptomatic. However, some patients develop significant neurologic sequelae, including encephalitis (generally indistinguishable from other forms of arboviral encephalitis,) and ascending flaccid paralysis similar to polio or Guillain–Barré syndrome.

   Diagnosis is based on serologic assessment of the blood or CSF. In symptomatic individuals, CSF generally demonstrates a lymphocytic pleocytosis and elevated protein. Treatment remains supportive.

CHRONIC MENINGITIS

Chronic meningitis presents with variable signs of meningeal irritation, cranial nerve dysfunction, and focal or global CNS dysfunction lasting 4 weeks or more. There is CSF pleocytosis, which may be caused by infectious or noninfectious processes (e.g., tuberculosis, fungus, hypersensitivity reaction, CNS tumor, chronic HIV, syphilis, and sarcoidosis). Treatment depends on the specific etiology.

BRAIN ABSCESS

If brain abscess is a consideration, avoid lumbar puncture until mass lesion has been excluded by CT or MRI. Aspiration or excision of brain abscesses, with appropriate antibiotic coverage and steroid therapy for edema, is the usual treatment. More conservative management of small abscesses with empiric antibiotics and close radiological follow-up is being used.

OTHER CENTRAL NERVOUS SYSTEM INFECTIONS

Lyme Disease

Lyme disease is a tick-borne spirochetal infection (caused by *Borrelia* species) with systemic and nervous system manifestations. Neurologic complications of early Lyme disease include:

1. Aseptic meningitis.
2. Cranial nerve palsies (especially facial nerve).
3. Mononeuritis multiplex.
4. Guillain-Barré syndrome.
5. Painful radiculoneuropathy.

Late-stage or chronic sequelae include sensory neuropathy, and, in rare cases, a chronic encephalopathy. Diagnosis may be difficult, and serology leads to overdiagnosis in endemic areas.

Patients with CNS complications of Lyme should have detectable antibodies in the serum and cerebrospinal fluid; the absence of antibodies makes the diagnosis highly unlikely.

Intravenous ceftriaxone (doses of 2 g/day for 2 to 4 weeks) is the therapy of choice for most neurologic complications of Lyme disease. Isolated facial nerve palsy, however, will respond adequately to oral doxycycline (if there is no evidence of CSF pleocytosis). Consider Lyme disease in a patient who has an unexplained meningitis, an unusual radiculopathy, Guillain–Barré syndrome, or an atypical facial palsy; especially when the typical rash or other key epidemiologic features (e.g., endemic area, tick bite) are present.

Repeated use of prolonged courses of antibiotics for so-called "chronic nervous system Lyme disease" has not been shown to improve long-term outcome in patients.

Neurosyphilis

Syphilis is associated with multiple neurologic complications. Invasion of the CNS during early syphilis may be associated with acute *meningitis*, but is often asymptomatic. In the absence of therapy, subacute or chronic meningitis may develop, accompanied by headache, cranial nerve palsies, seizures, and symptoms of increased intracranial pressure.

In *meningovascular syphilis*, strokes caused by vessel invasion occur.

In *tabes dorsalis*, there is inflammation of the dorsal roots and dorsal columns of the spinal cord, causing a sensory ataxia, bowel and bladder dysfunction, destruction of deafferented joints (Charcot joints), and episodes of severe, lancinating pains in the legs and body ("lightening pains"). Pupils are small, irregular, and reactive to accommodation, but not to light (Argyll–Robertson pupils), probably because of a partial third-nerve injury.

General paresis is a late manifestation of untreated syphilis with mental deterioration and occasional florid delusional ideas. Diagnosis is suggested by positive serologies (rapid plasma reagin [RPR] test, or Venereal Disease Research Laboratory [VDRL] test) and confirmed by fluorescent, treponemal antibody-absorption test (FTA-ABS) and an abnormal CSF. Treatment with penicillin is usually curative, but may not reverse neurologic deficits.

Cysticercosis

Found in endemic areas (primarily Latin America), cysticercosis is a parasitic infection of the brain with *Taenia solium* (larval form of the pork tapeworm). Symptoms include headache and seizure, with occasional obstructive hydrocephalus, or stroke. Cysticercosis affects 50 million people worldwide. Serologic testing may be diagnostic. CT scanning often shows multiple calcified lesions or focal areas of edema. Antihelminthics are key to definitive treatment. Standard antiepileptic medications are used for seizures.

Creutzfeld–Jakob Disease

This is a rare disorder due to an infectious protein (prion) affecting neuronal cells. CJD presents as a subacute progressive dementia sometimes with visual loss or motor neuron findings. This disease is untreatable and fatal. Most patients die within weeks; prolonged survival is rare. Electroencephalogram (EEG) may show characteristic periodic sharp waves. CSF may show 14-3-3 proteins as a marker, but recent studies have indicated that this is not specific for CJD. Brain biopsy may occasionally be needed, but puts health care workers at risk and positive diagnosis has no treatment options.

Listeria Rhombencephalitis

This is a rare condition with brainstem symptoms occurring in the setting of *Listeria* infection, with abnormal MRI and progressive neurologic dysfunction. A high index of suspicion, as well as CSF and blood cultures, is key in diagnosis.

Suggested Readings

DeGans J, van der Beek D. Dexamethasone in adults with bacterial meningitis. *N Engl J Med.* 2002;347:1549–1556.

Garcia HH, Del Brutto OH. Neurocysticercosis: updated concepts about an old disease. *Lancet Neurol.* 2005;4:653–661.

Kramer LD, Li J, Shi PY. West Nile virus. *Lancet Neurol.* 2007;6: 171–181.

Marra CM. Neurosyphilis: a guide for clinicians. *Neurologist.* 1995;1:157–166.

Steiner I, Budka H, Chaudhuri A, et al. Viral encephalitis: a review of diagnostic methods and guidelines for management. *Eur J Neurol.* 2005;12:331–343.

Wormser GP, Daddwyler RJ, Shapiro ED, et al. The clinical assessment, treatment, and prevention of Lyme disease, human granulocytic anaplasmosis, and babesiosis: clinical practice guidelines by the Infectious Diseases Society of America. *Clin Infect Dis.* 2006;43:1089–1134.

Wormser GP, Ramanathan R, Nowakowski J, et al. Duration of antibiotic therapy for early Lyme disease. A randomized, double-blind, placebo-controlled trial. *Ann Int Med.* 2003;138:697–704.

AIDS and the Nervous System

CASE

A 30-year-old woman with hemophilia develops a cough, shortness of breath, and has bilateral lung infiltrates on chest x-ray. She is also confused, with recent onset of right-sided weakness. MRI scanning of the brain with gadolinium shows multiple ring-enhancing lesions in both hemispheres with some mass effect. She is found to have a low CD4 count, tests positive for HIV virus, and a PCP pneumonia.

Diagnosis

Probable cerebral toxoplasmosis related to HIV/AIDS infection.

HIV NEUROLOGIC ISSUES

The nervous system is commonly affected by HIV virus-related disease. HIV-related neurologic symptoms can be caused by:

1. Direct infection of the nervous system.
2. Secondary opportunistic infections of the nervous system.
3. Tumors associated with AIDS.
4. Triggering of other processes (e.g., immune-mediated neuropathies).
5. Side effects of therapy for HIV, and related diseases.

No part of the nervous system is spared in patients with HIV infection. Areas of the nervous system that can be affected include:

1. Brain and brainstem.
2. Leptomeninges.
3. Spinal cord.
4. Peripheral nervous system.
5. Muscle.

The goal of the physician is to suspect and identify HIV infection in patients who have particular nervous system conditions, and to treat secondary infections accordingly. It is important to note that the use of highly active antiretroviral therapy (HAART) has markedly reduced the frequency of neurologic complications associated with HIV.

DIRECT INFECTION OF THE NERVOUS SYSTEM

HIV-Associated Dementia

Although many CNS manifestations of AIDS relate to secondary infections or tumors, the AIDS dementia complex is a specific clinical entity, caused by direct brain infection with HIV. Note the following:

1. Many patients with AIDS develop HIV-associated dementia (HAD). HAD usually develops after overt AIDS, although in many patients the dementia can present at the same time, or before other manifestations of AIDS.

   In some patients, dementia may be the only clinical sign of HIV infection at the time of diagnosis. HAD remains one of the most common causes of dementia in patients younger than age 40 years. Therefore, HIV testing should be included in the evaluation of a young patient with unexplained dementia.

2. The incidence of HAD has declined from approximately 21% to almost 10% in the era of combination antiretroviral therapy.

3. The onset of dementia is usually insidious, although some patients may experience an abrupt, rapid worsening of their condition, before sudden onset of dementia. In some patients, a rapidly accelerating dementia may occur in association with systemic illness.

4. Early symptoms and signs include:
   - Cognitive changes (including forgetfulness, mental slowing, and poor concentration).
   - Motor difficulties (ataxia, leg weakness, deteriorating handwriting).
   - Behavioral abnormalities (apathy, social withdrawal, psychosis).
   - Headache and seizures.

   Cortical features such as aphasia, apraxia, alexia, and agraphia are less common. Mild disturbances of eye movements are often present.

5. Late manifestations include severe dementia, ataxia, motor weakness, incontinence, tremor, mutism, and frontal release signs (e.g., rooting reflex and grasp response).

6. Some patients have an associated retinopathy, myelopathy, or peripheral neuropathy.

7. *Laboratory studies.* HAD typically occurs in the setting of moderately severe immunosuppression. Mean CD4 counts are usually below 200 mm^3. Cerebrospinal fluid (CSF) is abnormal in approximately half of the patients, and shows elevated protein levels, pleocytosis, and oligoclonal bands. Computed tomography (CT) or MRI scans are essential to rule out other focal conditions associated with AIDS (these conditions will be described later). Classic findings include atrophy, enlargement of cortical sulci, enlarged ventricles, and white-matter abnormalities. The detection of cerebral atrophy also has been reported among asymptomatic HIV patients, and is therefore not diagnostic of HAD. The electroencephalogram (EEG) is usually normal in the early stages of AIDS dementia complex.

8. Pathologic abnormalities result from direct viral invasion of the subcortical white matter, thalamus, and basal ganglia with relative sparing of the cerebral cortex. Neuron loss and astrocytosis are secondary effects of the viral invasion. An infiltration of macrophages is characteristic; these cells are believed to mediate much of the local damage via immunologic mechanisms. HAD is generally a diagnosis of exclusion.

   One must rule out other possible causes of dementia and delirium, including metabolic or drug-induced encephalopathy, cryptococcal meningitis, tuberculosis, intracranial mass lesion, neurosyphilis, encephalitis secondary to herpes simplex virus (HSV), varicella zoster virus (VZV), and cytomegalovirus (CMV).

9. Most experts recommend initiation of combination antiretroviral therapy in patients with HAD. Data demonstrating consistent improvements in HAD following therapy, unfortunately, are limited.

SECONDARY OPPORTUNISTIC INFECTIONS OF THE NERVOUS SYSTEM

Cerebral Toxoplasmosis

Cerebral toxoplasmosis is the most common cause of focal brain pathology (intracranial mass lesion) in patients with AIDS. It usually occurs when CD4+ counts are less than 100 cells/mm^3. It is important to recognize toxoplasmosis early, because prompt initiation of therapy can be successful.

Note the following:

1. *Presenting clinical symptoms* and signs include focal manifestations, most commonly hemiparesis. In addition, patients may have seizures, aphasia, cranial nerve palsies, and ataxia. The most common nonfocal manifestations are confusion, lethargy, and headache. Patients occasionally have parkinsonism or choreoathetosis as a result of lesions in the basal ganglia.
2. The most sensitive *laboratory studies* include MRI or CT scan, with contrast and blood serology. Ring-enhancing lesions are seen on both CT scan and MRI, although MRI imaging is more sensitive. Serum serologies almost always demonstrate elevated toxoplasma titers. Polymerase chain reaction (PCR) for toxoplasma in the CSF is sometimes helpful.
3. Most patients respond to *treatment* with pyrimethamine (200 mg initially followed by 75 mg PO daily) and sulfadiazine (1.5–2.0 g every 6 hours), if treated early. Leucovorin (10 to 20 mg PO daily) helps prevent pyrimethamine-associated bone marrow suppression. Clindamycin is recommended in place of sulfadiazine when patients report sulfa allergies. Steroids should be used only in patients with significant mass effect and edema. The duration of therapy is usually 6 weeks.
4. Because cerebral toxoplasmosis is one of the more treatable neurologic complications of AIDS, a therapeutic trial for toxoplasmosis is indicated before brain biopsy, in patients with suggestive radiographic findings and positive toxoplasma titers. Most patients demonstrate clinical and neuroradiographic improvement within 2 weeks of therapy. A failure to respond in 2 weeks warrants further diagnostic evaluation, which includes the possibility of stereotactic brain biopsy.

Other Infections of the Nervous System in HIV/AIDS

1. *Viral infections* include herpes simplex virus (HSV), varicella zoster virus (VZV), and cytomegalovirus (CMV), encephalitis, progressive multifocal leukoencephalopathy (PML—caused by the JC virus), and HIV or CMV retinitis. CMV retinitis can cause blindness, and can be treated with systemic ganciclovir, valganciclovir, foscarnet, or cidofovir. Intraocular ganciclovir implants or injections also may stabilize the disease. Aggressive treatment of HIV with combination antiretroviral therapy is essential to prevent recurrence of CMV

retinitis. An inflammatory vitritis may develop in patients with CMV retinitis who receive antiretroviral therapy as a result of immune reconstitution. The diagnosis of PML is supported by classic MRI findings (extensive, non-enhancing white matter disease), and the detection of JC virus in the CSF by the PCR.

2. *Nonviral infections* include tuberculosis, neurosyphilis, and fungal infections such as cryptococcus, *Candida*, and histoplasmosis.

TUMORS ASSOCIATED WITH AIDS

Neoplasms also affect the brain in patients with AIDS. The most common are primary central nervous system lymphoma, systemic lymphoma with CNS involvement, and Kaposi sarcoma.

Almost all primary CNS lymphomas are caused by Epstein–Barr virus in patients with advanced immunosuppression.

Most lesions are irregularly enhancing, and often deep in the brain in the corpus callosum. Many patients have confusion, lethargy, memory loss, hemiparesis. They may also have aphasia and seizures. Most have constitutional symptoms including fever, weight loss, and night sweats. CNS lymphoma is treated with radiation therapy and corticosteroids; many patients receive adjuvant chemotherapy. The prognosis of patients with CNS lymphoma and AIDS is often poor.

TRIGGERING OF OTHER PROCESSES

1. *Stroke*. In some patients, *infarction or hemorrhage* may occur. Hemorrhage may be associated with CNS lymphoma, and infarction may be the consequence of arteritis, endocarditis, meningovascular syphilis, or tuberculous vasculopathy.

2. Occasionally, immunologic-based diseases are triggered with HIV. These often occur early in the disease with seroconversion. Such diseases include acute inflammatory demyelinating polyneuropathy and mononeuritis multiplex.

SIDE EFFECTS OF THERAPY FOR HIV AND RELATED DISEASES

Drug-induced neuropathy: Some drugs used to treat AIDS such as didanosine (ddI), stavudine (d4T), and zalcitabine (ddC) may

■ **TABLE 25.1. Neurologic Complications in Patients Infected with HIV**

Brain

Predominantly nonfocal
  HIV-associated dementia
  CMV encephalitis
  Metabolic encephalopathies
  HSV encephalitis
  Acute HIV-1-related encephalitis
Predominantly focal
  Cerebral toxoplasmosis
  Primary CNS lymphoma
  Progressive multifocal leukoencephalopathy
  Cryptococcoma
  Varicella zoster virus encephalitis
  Tuberculous brain abscess/tuberculoma
  Neurosyphilis (meningovascular)
  Vascular disorders

Spinal cord

  Vacuolar myelopathy
  Herpes zoster myelitis
  HSV myelitis

Meninges

  Aseptic meningitis (HIV-1)
  Cryptococcal meningitis
  Metastatic lymphomatous meningitis
  Tuberculous meningitis
  Syphilitic meningitis

Peripheral nerve and root

Infectious
  Herpes zoster
  CMV polyradiculopathy
Virus or immune related
  Acute and chronic inflammatory demyelinating neuropathy
  Mononeuropathy
  Mononeuritis multiplex
  Autonomic neuropathy
  Sensorimotor polyneuropathy
  Distal painful sensory neuropathy

Muscle

  Polymyositis and other myopathies
  Drug-induced myopathies

cause a dose-related peripheral neuropathy. Discontinuation of the causative medication is essential for recovery. Antiretroviral-associated neuropathy is occasionally irreversible. An acute neuropathy associated with areflexia and ascending paresis has been associated with the development of lactic acidosis in patients treated with d4T and other antiretroviral medications. Mitochondrial damage is the postulated etiology for this condition (Table 25.1).

LOCALIZED CONDITIONS RELATED TO HIV OUTSIDE OF THE BRAIN

Leptomeninges

The leptomeninges frequently are involved in AIDS.

Examples of conditions occurring concurrently with AIDS are:

1. Cryptococcal meningitis.
2. Acute aseptic meningitis.
3. Lymphomatous meningitis.

Cryptococcal meningitis: Diagnosis of cryptococcal meningitis is based on lumbar puncture, CSF culture, and the detection of cryptococcal antigen in the serum and CSF. Symptoms include headache, confusion, and cranial nerve palsies. Patients may have sudden blindness due to increased intracranial pressure. Rapid diagnosis and treatment are key for survival. Patients may require CSF drainage to avoid secondary complication of increased intracranial pressure.

Acute "aseptic" meningitis: Patients present with headache, meningismus, cranial nerve palsies, and fever. This syndrome may occur at the time of seroconversion, and probably represents primary infection with HIV. This process is generally self-limited. In some instances, a more indolent form of HIV-related meningitis occurs, presenting only as headache and low-grade pleocytosis. Acute HIV should remain in the differential diagnosis of all patients (especially those with appropriate risk factors) who present with unexplained aseptic meningitis.

Lymphomatous meningitis: Systemic lymphoma may affect the meninges, and present with subacute systemic symptoms, headache, cranial nerve palsies, and confusion. MRI shows diffuse leptomeningeal enhancement. CSF shows a lymphocytic pleocytosis and cytology is key to the diagnosis.

Spinal Cord

1. Spinal cord involvement in AIDS includes vacuolar myelopathy from HIV infection and viral myelitis caused by HSV, VZV, and CMV, among others. These viral syndromes present with spinal cord dysfunction (e.g., leg weakness and incontinence) and increased cells in the spinal fluid.

2. A specific syndrome may be seen with CMV infection of the cauda equina, with a rapid onset of painful paraplegia and bowel and bladder dysfunction. PCR testing of the CSF may yield an early diagnosis of CMV, leading to successful therapy.

3. *Myelopathy associated with human T-lymphotrophic virus type 1 (HTLV-1).* A separate syndrome associated with HTLV-1 affects the spinal cord. It is unrelated to HIV infection, but is associated with another retrovirus, HTLV-1. This entity is termed tropical spastic paraparesis (TSP) or the HAM syndrome (HTLV-1-associated myelopathy). The HAM syndrome is endemic in southern Japan. Clinically, these patients have upper motor neuron spinal cord dysfunction associated with weakness, gait abnormalities, and spasticity. Patients also may have mild sensory and bladder disturbances. Diagnosis is based on elevated antibody titers to HTLV-1 virus in serum and spinal fluid. The cause of nervous system dysfunction is unclear. Treatment with steroids may be of temporary benefit. Danazol, interferon, and plasmapheresis also have been used with mixed results.

Peripheral Nerves

Peripheral nerve involvement may take the form of a sensory or sensorimotor polyneuropathy, inflammatory demyelinating polyneuropathy, mononeuropathy multiplex, and drug-related neuropathies.

1. *Sensory neuropathy* is seen in approximately 30% of patients. Symptoms include painful paresthesias affecting distal extremities. Symptoms occur late in the course of HIV infection. Treatment is symptomatic with drugs such as amitriptyline, nortriptyline, carbamazepine, gabapentin, or lamotrigine. Etiology is unclear and may relate to HIV infection of dorsal root ganglia plus nutritional and toxic factors.

2. *Inflammatory neuropathy* may be acute (Guillain–Barré syndrome), or chronic. In addition to increased CSF protein, these patients have significant CSF pleocytosis, which is generally not seen in typical cases of Guillain–Barré. Otherwise,

this syndrome may mimic Guillain–Barré syndrome, and may occur at HIV seroconversion. Patients respond to treatment with steroids or plasma exchange.

3. *Mononeuropathies* may be seen in HIV infection in association with the AIDS-related complex. Of patients with HIV infection, 5% to 10% will develop varicella zoster nerve root infection (radiculitis). The dermatomal rash is often diagnostic. Treatment with acyclovir, valacyclovir, or famciclovir is recommended. Postherpetic neuralgia is a possible complication.

Muscle

Myositis has been described as a complication of HIV infection. Muscle biopsies have shown inflammatory changes, including multinucleated giant cells, plus HIV antigens in the muscle. Treatment with steroids may be helpful. Myopathy also may be related to the therapy of HIV, especially zidovudine (AZT). Discontinuation of AZT typically leads to rapid improvement.

Suggested Readings

Carpenter CCJ, Cooper DA, Fischl MA, et al. Antiretroviral therapy in adults: updated recommendations of the international AIDS Society—USA Panel. *JAMA*. 2000;283:381–390.

d'Arminio MA, Duca PG, Vago L, et al. Decreasing incidence of CNS AIDS-defining events associated with antiretroviral therapy. *Neurology*. 2000;54:1856–1859.

Masur H, Kaplan JE, Holmes KK, et al. Recommendations of the U.S. Public Health Service and the Infectious Diseases Society of America. *Ann Intern Med*. 2002;137:435–478.

Treisman GJ, Kaplin AI. Neurologic and psychiatric complications of antiretroviral agents. *AIDS*. 2002;16:1201–1215.

Neurology of Uremia

CASE

A 64-year-old man with end-stage renal failure tells you that at night his legs "bother him." Just after he lies down in bed, his legs feel "odd," and he has to get up and walk. He can't quite put the feeling into words, but it keeps him from having a restful sleep.

Diagnosis

Restless leg syndrome, associated with renal disease.

Patients with impaired renal function have a variety of neurologic problems. They are at a higher risk of mental status changes, peripheral neuropathy, neurologic infection, and other manifestations of their underlying disease state.

MENTAL STATUS CHANGES

One of the most common features of renal failure is an altered mental status. It may range from irritability and difficulty concentrating (e.g., performing "serial 7s"), to psychotic reactions or coma.

Mental status changes in uremia fluctuate; periods of confusion are interspersed with periods of lucidity. *Acute changes in mental status* generally are encountered after dialysis, when there have been rapid electrolyte shifts; although actual electrolyte values are improved ("dysequilibrium syndrome"). Metabolic shifts in brain pH or urea often lag behind the changes in the blood values. Slowly developing renal failure causes fewer cognitive changes than does rapidly developing failure. Acute uremia may be accompanied by tremor, fasciculations, myoclonus, chorea, or convulsions. Patients undergoing dialysis are at risk for complex partial status epilepticus, and patients with an unexplained encephalopathy should have an electroencephalogram (EEG).

EEG changes are usual with an altered mental status, and *slowing* usually parallels the degree of metabolic encephalopathy.

Most patients with a blood urea nitrogen level higher than 60 mg/100 mL have EEG abnormalities (*generalized slowing*). With complex partial status, continuous focal seizure activity or rhythmic slowing may be seen.

Although most mental status changes in uremia are not secondary to treatable nervous system disease, keep other possibilities in mind:

1. *Infection.* Listeria, fungal, or other central nervous system (CNS) pathogens are not uncommon in patients with uremia. When there is unexplained confusion or fever in the patient with uremia, after performing a CT scan or magnetic resonance imaging (MRI) to rule out subdural hematoma or other mass lesion, perform a lumbar puncture (LP). Remember to do an India ink preparation for *Cryptococcus* or test for cryptococcal antigen if there are cells in the cerebrospinal fluid (CSF) (see Chapter 30).

2. *Subdural hematoma.* Patients with uremia have an increased bleeding tendency, and subdural collections may develop with mild head trauma or during dialysis. If a subdural hematoma is suspected because of lateralizing signs or persistent lethargy with headache, obtain a CT or MRI scan.

3. *Hypertensive encephalopathy.* Hypertension frequently accompanies uremia, and hypertensive crisis may mimic the clinical features of uremic encephalopathy. Look for markedly elevated blood pressure, papilledema, and retinal hemorrhages. MRI changes that are bilateral, subcortical, and suggestive of edema may be dramatic, and are reversible with resolution of the hypertensive encephalopathy. Patients with cyclosporine toxicity may be especially sensitive to mild hypertension, which can cause a reversible posterior hemisphere leukoencephalopathy (otherwise known as PRESS, posterior reversible encephalopathy syndrome). Clinically, these patients present with confusion, lethargy, and visual symptoms. They respond to lowering blood pressure and withholding cyclosporine.

SEIZURES

Seizures are a common feature of renal disease. They signify different processes, depending on the type (generalized or focal), and the clinical setting (e.g., postdialysis). Patients with acute anuria may develop tonic-clonic seizures on the 8th to 11th day of renal failure, or with the onset of diuresis, and subsequent rapid electrolyte shifts.

Tonic-clonic seizures also appear late in the course of *chronic renal disease*, and frequently are associated with abnormal blood chemistries; these being acidosis, hypokalemia, and hyponatremia. No one abnormal electrolyte is associated consistently with seizures.

Remember, generalized tonic-clonic seizures caused by metabolic disorders may not respond to antiepileptic drugs; consider dialysis and aggressive management of the metabolic abnormalities. This is especially important when status epilepticus is present.

PERIPHERAL NEUROPATHY

1. *Early*

   Patients often develop a "restless leg syndrome" as an early sign of uremic neuropathy. The legs feel uncomfortable when the patient is still, and relief occurs after ambulation. Another early neuropathic syndrome consists of painful, burning paresthesias of the feet similar to those seen in alcoholics and associated with dietary insufficiency. Resolution may follow proper diet and vitamin supplements.

2. *Late*

   A more severe peripheral neuropathy develops over weeks to months, and is not diet-dependent. Check for distal loss of all sensory modalities (pinprick, position, vibration). The legs are affected significantly more than the arms. The neuropathy is motor and sensory, and may lead to actual paraplegia (at this stage the arms also may become involved). Treatment is difficult.

OTHER NEUROLOGIC FEATURES OF UREMIA

Dialysis may precipitate convulsions, or a toxic encephalopathy. In this "reverse urea syndrome," urea leaves the brain more slowly than it leaves the blood; fluid, thus, is drawn into the brain, resulting in acute swelling. The encephalopathy usually clears in 24 to 48 hours. Remember, subdural hematoma sometimes follows dialysis.

1. *Asterixis* frequently accompanies uremic encephalopathy; as do muscle fasciculations and myoclonus.

2. *Muscle cramps* may occur, and generally are unrelated to a specific electrolyte abnormality; although they are more frequent when water intoxication is present.

3. Chvostek sign may be positive in uremia; it is correlated with the acidosis and elevated potassium/calcium ratio, rather than with decreased calcium alone. There may be mild proximal muscle weakness.

4. *Uremic amaurosis* has been reported with the acute development of blindness; this may be related to focal cerebral edema. Complete recovery usually occurs.

5. *Cerebral emboli* may occur during the declotting of shunts used for hemodialysis.

6. *Dialysis dementia* has been reported in patients with uremia; it represents a subacutely progressive neurologic deterioration in patients undergoing hemodialysis.

    It consists of:
    • Dementia.
    • Myoclonus.
    • Speech disorders.
    • Neuropsychiatric abnormalities.
    • Gait abnormalities.
    • EEG changes (periodic sharp waves or spike and wave).

7. Aluminum intoxication appears to be an important factor. Clinical and EEG improvement may follow treatment with diazepam, or other anticonvulsants. This disorder has become rarer with removal of aluminum from most dialysate solutions.

    Note that patients with renal failure on penicillins or cephalosporins may develop confusion, myoclonus, seizures, and coma. Reduction or withdrawal of the offending agents is the treatment.

8. Gabapentin in renal failure patients may cause the same syndrome, if not dose adjusted for the level of renal dysfunction.

9. *Carpal tunnel syndrome* is common in patients undergoing hemodialysis. Focal neuropathies sometimes are associated with vascular graft placement, occurring distal to the graft site, and are related to vascular steal phenomena as a result of the graft.

10. Uremic myopathy may occur. This is often associated with bone pain and tenderness, and is similar to that found in primary hyperparathyroidism and osteomalacia.

Suggested Readings

Bruno A, Adams HP. Neurologic problems in renal transplant recipients. *Neurol Clin.*1989;7:617–627.

Burn DJ, Bates D. Neurology and the kidney. *J Neurol Neurosurg Psychiatry.* 1998;65:810–821.

De Deyn PP, Saxena VK, Abts H, et al. Clinical and pathophysiological aspects of neurological complications in renal failure. *Acta Neurol Belgica*. 1992;92:191–206.

Smogorzewski MJ. Central nervous dysfunction in uremia. *Am J Kidney Dis*. 2001;38(suppl 1):S122–S128.

Neurology
of Alcoholism

CASE

The chief executive officer of a small company is admitted for an appendectomy. Two days postsurgery, he experiences two generalized tonic-clonic seizures that occur within 15 minutes of each other. The patient is jittery, anxious, and sweating, with a moderate tachycardia. He admits that he drinks three large Manhattans every night, and more on weekends. Results of an electroencephalogram (EEG) and magnetic resonance imaging scan with gadolinium are normal.

Diagnosis

Alcohol withdrawal seizures.

SEIZURES

Seizures are common in the person who is an alcoholic, and represent at least two different phenomena. It is important to distinguish the two types of "alcoholic seizures," because treatment and workup are different.

Alcoholic Withdrawal Seizures

Alcoholic withdrawal seizures are brief, self-limited, generalized seizures secondary to abstinence from alcohol, or a reduction in the usual intake. They do not represent a true convulsive disorder and most occur 12 to 48 hours after cessation of drinking (rarely after 96 hours). Remember, alcohol withdrawal seizures can occur in the "businessman drinker" who comes to the hospital for other reasons; often for an operation. Alcohol withdrawal seizures tend to appear in groups of two or three, and then stop. The patient is usually tremulous and jittery. The interictal EEG in these patients is usually normal, and if the history is characteristic, the patient requires no further neurologic workup, or anticonvulsant medication. Standard treatment for alcohol withdrawal is sufficient. A subgroup of alcoholics has seizures for other reasons, such as subdural hemotoma, head injury, and the like.

Some imaging study is probably important in alcoholics with seizures.

Patients with alcoholic withdrawal seizures are also at a higher risk for developing delirium tremens (DTs).

ALCOHOLIC TREMULOUSNESS— DELIRIUM TREMENS (DTS)

The spectrum of alcohol withdrawal symptoms ranges from mild tremulousness to fatal DTs. The underlying physiology in these states is related to abstinence from alcohol, not to specific dietary or vitamin insufficiency. Similar withdrawal states can occur after stopping other central nervous system (CNS) depressants (e.g., barbiturates, diazepam). DTs and withdrawal seizures can be produced in normal people with good diets who are placed on large amounts of alcohol, and then withdrawn. Seizures are a point on the spectrum of withdrawal symptomatology. An alcoholic who stops drinking is subject to the following:

1. *Tremulousness* is one of the first signs of alcohol withdrawal; beginning approximately 8 hours after cessation of drinking (often after a night's sleep), and reaching its peak at 24 hours. The patient is jittery, startles easily, and often shows a gross irregular tremor of the hands. There are signs of sympathetic overactivity, with increased sweating and heart rate. Although these symptoms are most severe at 24 hours, it may take 7 to 10 days before the patient is back to normal.
2. *Seizures* (discussed earlier).
3. *Hallucinations* appear during the withdrawal period and are commonly visual, although they may be auditory. Sometimes the patient hallucinates in the presence of an otherwise clear sensorium.
4. *DTs* complete the spectrum. This serious reaction occurs approximately 72 to 96 hours after cessation of drinking. Patients suffer from tremulousness, hallucinations, and marked autonomic hyperactivity (tachycardia, hyperhidrosis, fever, dilated pupils).

   DTs are a relatively uncommon sequelae of alcoholic withdrawal, but can be fatal; they often are preceded by an alcoholic withdrawal seizure. The mortality rate is significant if

DTs are untreated, because of cardiovascular collapse, self-injury, electrolyte disorders, and infections.

Treatment of Delirium Tremens

Treatment consists primarily of supportive care. Adequate diet and vitamins have no effect on the course of alcohol withdrawal, but must be given to prevent other complications.

Pay careful attention to fluid and electrolyte balance (several liters of saline a day may be needed), correct hypoglycemia, and search thoroughly for underlying disease (e.g., subdural hematoma, pneumonia, or meningitis).

These diseases are not uncommon, and often are the factors that make DTs fatal. Treat with diazepam, 10 mg intravenously (IV), then 5 mg or more every 5 minutes up to 40 mg IV until the patient is calm with maintenance of 5 mg or more IV or intramuscularly (IM) every 1 to 4 hours as needed. Other benzodiazepines; such as lorazepam and chlordiazepoxide, also may be used. There is no evidence that steroids are of benefit. Atenolol, a beta-adrenergic blocker, is sometimes helpful in selected patients with the alcohol withdrawal syndrome.

VITAMIN DEFICIENCY SYNDROMES AND ALCOHOLISM

In addition to the alcohol withdrawal syndrome, there is a group of vitamin deficiency syndromes seen almost exclusively in alcoholics. These also appear in nonalcoholics with poor diets, or with cachexia associated with cancer.

Wernicke Encephalopathy

Wernicke encephalopathy is an important deficiency disorder, caused by a lack of thiamine, which is associated with changes in the thalamus and brainstem. It causes a classic triad:

1. *Oculomotor changes.* Look for nystagmus on horizontal or vertical gaze, sixth-nerve palsies that are generally bilateral, and paralysis of conjugate gaze. In severe forms, there may be total ophthalmoplegia.
2. *Gait difficulties.* Check for ataxia: a wide-based gait, falling, or inability to walk or stand. Limb ataxia (finger-to-arm testing) is usually absent.

3. *Mental symptoms*. Patients usually manifest a quiet, apathetic, confused state. *Korsakoff psychosis* is an extension of the mental symptoms of Wernicke disease, and becomes apparent later if the Wernicke syndrome is untreated. The main feature is a marked disorder of memory with confabulation.

Remember, Wernicke encephalopathy often is under-diagnosed, and may not present with all parts of the classic triad. Consider Wernicke encephalopathy in confused patients who have nutritional deficiencies of any type. Treat early and aggressively. In addition to the previously mentioned triad, thiamine deficiency can produce dysautonomia, including cardiac failure, and electrocardiography abnormalities.

Treatment consists of thiamine (100 mg IV diluted in 100 mL of normal saline, or D5% given over ½ hour) to improve the oculomotor dysfunction, and to prevent the development of Korsakoff psychosis. Gastrointestinal malabsorption in alcoholics makes oral treatment unreliable. A 50-mg IM dose should be repeated daily, until the patient resumes a normal diet.

Wernicke syndrome also can occur in nonalcoholics who depend on parenteral alimentation (e.g., surgical or burn unit patients). It can also be seen in patients with malnutrition as a result of starvation, renal failure, cancer, or acquired immune deficiency syndrome.

Polyneuropathy

Polyneuropathy occurs in alcoholics secondary to nutritional factors, and also may be related in part to the toxic effects of alcohol. Most patients are asymptomatic, but lose ankle and sometimes knee jerks. When symptoms occur, they consist of burning, painful feet, with mild distal weakness. The feet may be so sensitive that even the touch of the bed covers is painful. In severe cases, the weakness may progress to wrist-drop and foot-drop. Polyneuropathy and Wernicke syndrome often occur in the same patient.

Treatment consists of improving the diet, completely abstaining from alcohol, and adding vitamin supplements.

OTHER NEUROLOGIC COMPLICATIONS OF ALCOHOLISM

Cerebellar degeneration affects men more frequently than women, and midline structures more than the cerebellar hemispheres. Thus, there is a wide-based gait with truncal instability, and less prominent limb ataxia. The symptoms appear over weeks to months, although they may come on acutely. The acutely occurring syndrome has a better prognosis, and may not represent actual cerebellar structural damage; as does the chronic form. Treatment consists of dietary and vitamin support.

Abstinence from alcohol is crucial.

Some patients may have slowly developing myopathy with proximal muscle weakness, often in conjunction with alcoholic cardiac myopathy. There is an acute form with muscle pain, weakness, and elevated creatinine phosphokinase and myoglobinuria. Treatment is symptomatic. Rare complications of alcoholism or malnutrition include *central pontine myelinolysis* and the *Marchiafava–Bignami corpus callosum syndrome*.

NEUROLOGIC COMPLICATIONS OF OTHER DRUGS

The neurologic complications of drugs other than alcohol are beyond the scope of this text. A few points about other drugs are as follows:

1. Opioids cause euphoria, sedation, nausea, sweating, constipation, and analgesia. They also cause miosis, which is a useful sign. Overdose causes coma, respiratory depression, and pinpoint, but reactive pupils.
2. Stimulant medications such as amphetamines and cocaine cause increased motor activity and physical endurance. Overdose may cause hypertension, tachycardia, headache, chest pain, and fever. Delirium, cardiac arrhythmias, seizures, and strokes may occur.
3. Sedative agents such as barbiturates and benzodiazepines cause sedation and respiratory suppression. Withdrawal of such agents may cause seizures, tremors, and agitation, all of which may be suppressed by the institution of barbiturate or benzodiazepines.
4. Marijuana causes a euphoric state, disinhibition, and postural hypotension. Fatal overdose has not been reported.
5. Hallucinogens such as lysergic acid diethylamide cause perceptual distortions, hallucinosis, and sense of depersonalization. Some patients experience "flashbacks." There are vivid recurrence of drug symptoms long after the cessation of drug use.
6. Glue sniffing and use of other inhalants, such as lighter fluid, cause symptoms such as euphoria, somnolence, hallucinations, and seizures.
7. Phencyclidine (PCP) causes stimulant symptoms; in addition to paranoia, hallucinosis, rhabdomyolysis, and seizures. Symptoms can persist for hours to days.

Suggested Readings

Bayard M, McIntyre J, Hill KR, et al. Alcohol withdrawal syndrome. *Am Fam Physician*. 2004;69:1443–1450.

Mayo-Smith MF, Beecher LH, et al. Management of alcohol withdrawal delirium. An evidence-based practice guideline. *Arch Intern Med*. 2004;164:1405–1412.

O'Connor PG, Schottenfeld RS. Patients with alcohol problems. *N Engl J Med*. 1998;338:592–602.

Sechi G, Serra A. Wernicke's encephalopathy: new clinical settings and recent advances in diagnosis and management. *Lancet Neurol*. 2007;6:442–455.

Neurology of Other Systemic Diseases

CASE

A 57-year-old woman complains of weakness when getting out of a chair, and a hoarse voice. She has been losing hair and gaining weight, and friends tell her she is "slowing down." On examination, her reflexes are hypoactive, and her muscles feel doughy to the touch.

Diagnosis

Hypothyroidism with myopathy and neuropathy.

Many systemic diseases exhibit neurologic manifestations. This has been described in preceding chapters regarding the neurology of diabetes, malignancy, uremia, and alcohol, as well as in the stroke chapter. The physician must recognize the many neurologic complications that accompany systemic disorders and treat them accordingly.

CARDIAC DISEASE

Cardiac abnormalities can cause reduced cerebral perfusion, or emboli that lead to neurologic sequelae. The severity of neurologic manifestations of reduced cardiac output varies with the rate and extent of decreased cerebral perfusion.

Ischemic brain injury can lead to seizures, cerebral edema, loss of consciousness, amnesia, and dementia.

Emboli from the heart are the cause of 15% of ischemic strokes. Thrombi, from which emboli emerge, may develop from a left atrial or ventricular mural thrombus, an intracardiac tumor, bacterial and nonbacterial endocarditis, or the systemic and right heart circulation via intracardiac shunts (paradoxic emboli).

Conditions that predispose the patient to develop such emboli include:

1. Atrial fibrillation.
2. Acute and chronic ischemic heart disease.
3. Valvular heart diseases (rheumatic and prosthetic).

Patent foramen ovale and atrial septal aneurysm also can cause cerebral emboli. The role of closure of patent foramen ovale is still being reevaluated at the present time.

Patients with recurrent emboli who have no other cause of embolism other than PFO are candidates for catheter closure of PFO. Some of these patients have associated coagulation disorders and should be evaluated for such disorders.

Young patients with strokes, but without evidence of cerebrovascular disease, should still be suspected of having a cardiac cause of stroke.

Electrocardiogram (ECG), echocardiography, prolonged ECG monitoring to identify arrhythmias, and transesophageal echocardiography are helpful tests for detecting the cause of cardiogenic stroke. Transthoracic echocardiography has a low yield in showing cardiac sources of embolism, and is not an effective "screening tool" for embolic sources of stroke.

Anticoagulation therapy reduces the risk of embolism in atrial fibrillation, rheumatic mitral stenosis, and cardiomyopathy with ventricular thrombi.

After a myocardial infarction (MI), patients are at risk for stroke, especially with anterior wall infarction. If echocardiography detects a developing thrombus, anticoagulation reduces the risk of post-MI stroke by at least 60%.

Anoxic encephalopathy, lack of oxygen to the brain, often occurs in the setting of cardiac arrest. Mild degrees of hypoxemia cause inattention, drowsiness, and impaired judgment. In patients with prior deficits, hypoxemia may make symptoms worse.

Anoxic injury may cause a variety of symptoms that can occur individually or in combination and include the following:

1. Cortical damage or a watershed infarction, leading to dementia or visual agnosia.
2. Cerebellar injury, causing ataxia and/or action myoclonus.
3. Memory impairment caused by injury to the mesial thalamus and hippocampus.
4. Choreoathetosis or a parkinsonian syndrome.
5. "Man in the barrel" syndrome; with weakness of shoulder girdle muscles sparing the hands, so the affected person cannot abduct the arms. This pattern results from infarction affecting the shoulder region in the cortex, which lies between anterior and middle cerebral territories in the watershed zone.
6. Coma, stupor, or persistent vegetative state may occur with severe diffuse injury.

Recently cooling of body temperature, beginning within 6 hours of an anoxic event, has been shown to significantly improve

functional outcome and survival. This should be considered in any patient who is not immediately awakening after an anoxic event.

Cardiac complications of open heart surgery are a major source of morbidity in the postoperative state. These include both central nervous system complications and peripheral nervous system disorders. The four following disorders are the most common neurologic problems after open heart surgery:

1. *Encephalopathy:* A generalized encephalopathy occurs in about 6% of patients after open heart surgery. This is more common with elderly patients, prolonged surgery, a patient with preexisting cognitive dysfunction, and patients with major underlying medical morbidities, such as renal failure. This usually improves. When measured, however, many patients post open heart surgery have some level of cognitive decline.

2. *Stroke:* Stroke syndromes are a major source of morbidity after open heart surgery and occur in about 3% to 5% of open heart surgery patients. Most of these are due to emboli from the arch, microemboli from cardiac bypass, or due to atrial fibrillation, and are not usually related to carotid atherosclerosis. Stroke is more common in patients undergoing valvular surgery than patients having coronary artery bypass grafting. It is unclear whether surgery or stenting for severe carotid stenosis prior to open heart surgery is beneficial, as there are no randomized trials of these treatments.

3. *Anoxic encephalopathy:* Anoxic encephalopathy can occur with open heart surgery, and is usually associated with documented severe hypotension, or cessation of circulation other than the usual bypass transitions.

4. *Brachial plexopathy:* Between 2% and 10% of post open heart patients will develop a brachial plexopathy. This appears to be due to injury to the brachial plexus by compression from the dorsal ribs, rather than from stretch injury (anatomic studies). It may cause burning pain in an arm; usually in a lower trunk distribution causing tingling and burning in the fifth digits, and weakness of intrinsic hand muscles. It may improve slowly if at all.

ENDOCRINE DISEASE

1. *Thyroid disease:* Hyperthyroid patients often complain of anxiety, fatigue, and irritability. They may have seizures, tremor, chorea, and usually have brisk tendon reflexes. They also may develop ophthalmopathy, including proptosis and

ophthalmoplegia. A myopathy with proximal muscle weakness and wasting is not uncommon. On physical examination, hypoactive reflexes with a delayed relaxation time usually can be demonstrated. Reflexes may be pendular (i.e., the leg swings to and fro more often than normal if allowed to swing freely). Encephalopathy may occur with Hashimoto thyroiditis. In this syndrome patients may have confusion, altered consciousness, and seizures associated with increased anti-thyroid antibodies, and may respond to steroid therapy. Myxedema coma is rare and carries a high mortality rate. Some myxedematous patients may develop seizures, obstructive sleep apnea, ataxia, or sensorineural hearing loss.

   Note: **Check for hyperthyroidism in patients with action tremor; check for hypothyroidism in patients with carpal tunnel syndrome.**

2. *Parathyroid:* Patients with *hyperparathyroidism* often display psychiatric symptoms, such as those associated with mania, schizophrenia, or depression. Myopathy is common. Patients with hypoparathyroidism may have psychiatric symptoms similar to those seen in *hyperparathyroidism*. Seizures can occur from hypocalcemia; particularly in hyperparathyroid patients after adenoma removal. Hypocalcemia and hypomagnesemia can cause tetany. To elicit latent tetany, have the patient hyperventilate and tap the facial nerve, causing facial muscle contraction (Chvostek sign), or occlude venous return from an arm, resulting in carpopedal spasm (Trousseau sign). Laryngeal spasm also may occur in this setting.

3. *Glucocorticoids:* Myopathy is common with corticosteroid therapy, and myalgia may accompany the weakness. Treatment involves tapering or use of alternate-day steroids, alternate forms of immunosuppression, or nonfluorinated steroids. Patients with Cushing syndrome may experience psychiatric symptoms, and occasionally frank psychosis. Patients on exogenous steroids may also experience such symptoms, as well as insomnia. Patients with Addison disease, and patients after withdrawal from steroids, may experience acute confusional states or psychosis. Seizures can occur from hyponatremia.

FLUID AND ELECTROLYTE DISTURBANCES

1. *Sodium:* Manifestations of *hyponatremia* range from confusion to coma.

Patients also may experience:
- Convulsions.
- Hemiparesis.
- Ataxia, tremor.
- Aphasia.
- Corticospinal tract signs.

Sodium must be corrected to 120 to 125 mEq/L when convulsions are present, because such patients have a high mortality if this is not done. However, too rapid correction of hyponatremia may result in central pontine myelinolysis.

Central pontine myelinolysis: a subacute demyelinating disorder in response to rapid electrolyte changes with changes in the pons and midbrain. Patients may develop quadriparesis, dysphagia, and altered mental status.

2. *Potassium: Hypokalemia* causes muscle weakness, myalgia, and fatigability. With very low potassium levels (less than 2.5 mEq/L), rhabdomyolysis and myoglobinuria may occur. Rapid recovery occurs with potassium replacement. Occasionally, this state is mistaken for Guillain–Barré syndrome. *Hyperkalemia* is cardiotoxic, and rarely is associated with neurologic symptoms before the heart is affected.

3. *Calcium: Hypercalcemia* may occur in patients with malignant neoplasms (particularly breast and lung cancer and multiple myeloma), and in patients with hyperparathyroidism. Patients may experience:
- Lethargy.
- Muscle weakness.
- Fatigability.
- Confusion.
- Headache.
- Convulsions.
- Coma.

Hypocalcemia is less common, but is seen in patients with renal failure. Acute hypocalcemia most often occurs after thyroid or parathyroid surgery, and is a complication of acute pancreatitis. Patients are agitated and may experience delirium, hallucinations, and psychosis. Seizures may occur. Hypocalcemia (or hypomagnesemia) can cause tetany.

4. *Magnesium*: With decreased magnesium, patients are irritable and confused and may experience tetany, convulsions, tremor, and myoclonus. They are hyper-reflexic and demonstrate a Chvostek sign. Treatment of convulsions is with parental magnesium. *Hypermagnesemia* is rare and occurs with increased

intake in the setting of decreased renal function. It causes lethargy and confusion, and muscle paralysis may result.

GASTROINTESTINAL DISEASE

1. *Hepatic encephalopathy:* Mental changes range from delirium to coma. Tremor, paratonia, asterixis, and hyperactive reflexes also are seen.

   Asterixis is a sudden cessation of muscle activity, and is best seen by having the patient hold the hands extended at the wrists with the arms outstretched. The hands suddenly fall forward, and then rise up again. It also may be seen in other metabolic disorders, or with drug intoxications. The electroencephalogram (EEG) demonstrates slowing and triphasic waves. Serum ammonia levels may be increased, but do not correlate well with the presence of hepatic encephalopathy.

   Causes of encephalopathy include toxins and metabolic derangements.

   Gastrointestinal (GI) bleeding frequently precipitates hepatic encephalopathy. If focal neurologic symptoms occur in the setting of hepatic encephalopathy, look for a structural lesion. Hepatic encephalopathy may unmask previously asymptomatic lesions, such as a chronic subdural hematoma. Imaging also may demonstrate subarachnoid or intracerebral hemorrhage, related to coagulopathy associated with hepatic disease. Antibiotics (e.g., neomycin oral) appeared to be superior to non-absorbable disaccharides in improving hepatic encephalopathy, but there is limited high-quality evidence about the treatment of hepatic encephalopathy.

2. *Malabsorption:* Several GI disorders are associated with malabsorption (e.g., inflammatory bowel disease, postgastric resection).

   This may lead to thiamine deficiency, Wernicke encephalopathy, or Korsakoff psychosis (see Chapter 27).

   Cyanocobalamin (vitamin B_{12}) can be deficient in a vegetarian's diet, after gastric resection, with intrinsic factor deficiency (pernicious anemia), in a patient without a functional terminal ileum, or with pancreatic insufficiency. Patients experience paresthesias, sensory loss, ataxia, and dementia.

   Patients who lack vitamin B_6 can develop peripheral neuropathy. Those with vitamin A deficiency have an increased risk of night blindness; inadequate amounts of vitamin E cause neuropathy and cerebellar dysfunction. There are recent reports of "swayback"; a spinal cord syndrome due to copper deficiency, occurring in the gastric bypass population.

Watch out for neurologic complications of gastric bypass surgery due to malabsorption of vitamins and trace metals.

3. *Wilson disease: Wilson disease* is an autosomal recessive disorder of copper metabolism manifested by cirrhosis, and degeneration of the caudate and putamen.

   Medical complications include hepatic dysfunction, and an autoimmune hemolytic anemia. Patients may have tremor, dysarthria, dementia, and psychiatric symptoms.

   Patients have a Kayser–Fleischer ring on ophthalmologic examination, decreased serum ceruloplasmin level, and increased copper concentration on liver biopsy.

4. *Other disorders: Chronic hepatocerebral degeneration* is a slowly progressive neurologic syndrome, manifested by chronic intermittent episodes of hepatic encephalopathy, and seen in patients with hepatic disease. Permanent neurologic signs and symptoms may result, including:
   • Tremor.
   • Ataxia.
   • Dysarthria.
   • Nystagmus.
   • Dementia.
   • Choreoathetosis.
   • Pyramidal tract signs.
   • Grasp reflexes.

Patients with portal–systemic shunts may experience a myelopathy associated with dysarthria. The etiology is unclear.

Note: Inflammatory bowel disease may be associated with several neurologic problems, including peripheral neuropathies, myelopathy, myopathy, myasthenia, and cerebrovascular disorders. *Whipple disease* may cause an encephalopathy, and occasionally a movement disorder called oculomyorhythmia, with oscillatory eye and mouth movements.

HEMATOLOGIC DISEASE

1. *Anemia:* Common symptoms of anemia include fatigue, headache, and lightheadedness. Individuals with sickle-cell anemia may develop stroke, convulsions, or a change in level of consciousness. Patients with chronic hematologic diseases, characterized by bone marrow failure or hemolytic anemia, have extramedullary hematopoiesis that may involve meninges

surrounding the spinal cord and brain, leading to myelopathy or intracranial mass lesions.

2. *Hyperviscosity:* Patients with hyperviscosity may experience headache, lightheadedness, tinnitus, stupor, convulsions, or stroke. Causative diseases include polycythemia vera, leukocytosis, and paraproteinemias with Waldenström macroglobulinemia, and multiple myeloma. Patients with leukemia have a high incidence of intracerebral hemorrhage, and patients with paraproteinemia have reduced cerebral blood flow, peripheral neuropathies, mononeuritis multiplex, and cerebral infarction.

3. *Thrombocytopenia:* Immune thrombocytopenic purpura can follow viral infection, with an increased incidence of intracranial hemorrhage. Patients with thrombotic thrombocytopenic purpura have prominent neurologic symptoms including headache, hemiparesis, aphasia, and seizures. Corticosteroids and plasma exchange are of benefit in treatment.

4. *Hemophilia:* Patients with hemophilia are predisposed to develop intracranial hemorrhage, subdural hematoma, subarachnoid hemorrhage, and epidural hematoma of the spinal cord. Peripheral neuropathies may develop secondary to compression, by soft-tissue hemorrhage; particularly femoral neuropathy from retroperitoneal bleeding. These bleeding complications also may occur in patients receiving anticoagulation therapy.

5. Paraproteinemias may be associated with a variety of peripheral nerve disorders. Some of these may respond to immunologic therapies, such as plasmapheresis and steroid therapy.

6. Antiphospholipid antibodies, including lupus anticoagulant and anticardiolipin antibodies, may be associated with focal cerebral ischemia, and should be tested for in young patients with unexplained cerebral ischemic events. There is a variable relationship between the presence of these antibodies, and other collagen vascular disorders such as lupus. Cardiac disease (e.g., marantic endocarditis) often underlies the stroke syndromes in such patients.

PULMONARY DISEASE

1. *Respiratory insufficiency:* Hypoxia, hypercapnia, and respiratory acidosis may cause headache, mental status changes, motor disturbances, ocular abnormalities, and paresthesias. Twitching and tremor result from increased sympathetic nervous system activity. Asterixis, generalized seizures, and myoclonus may occur. Polycythemia from chronic respiratory insufficiency causes headache and dizziness.

2. *Hyperventilation:* Anxious individuals may have neurologic symptoms, including paresthesias if they hyperventilate, light-headedness, altered consciousness, carpal spasm, muscle cramps, visual blurring, dyspnea, chest pain, and an elicitable Chvostek sign. Hyperventilation syndrome is usually psychogenic, but it may be associated with medication, alcohol withdrawal, or central nervous system (CNS) lesions. Rebreathing into a paper bag at the first awareness of symptoms, and taking beta blockers may be helpful.

RHEUMATOLOGIC DISEASES, SARCOIDOSIS, AND VASCULITIDES

1. *Systemic lupus erythematosus (SLE):* Half of patients with lupus have neurologic manifestations, but most have an established diagnosis of SLE, before neurologic manifestations develop. Central nervous system (CNS) lupus includes strokes, seizures, ataxia, chorea, meningitis, cranial neuropathies, and optic neuritis. CNS lupus is usually due to vascular disease of the brain, and is usually not a "vasculitis" per se. It is usually treated with corticosteroids, cyclophosphamide, azathioprine, or plasmapheresis.

   CNS infections are more frequent in patients with lupus, because of immunosuppressive therapy. Psychotropic medications may provide symptomatic relief of neuropsychiatric manifestations. The peripheral nervous system (PNS) is affected less frequently than the CNS, but patients may have sensory and sensorimotor neuropathies, mononeuropathies, mononeuritis multiplex, and an acute ascending sensorimotor neuropathy similar to Guillain–Barré syndrome.

2. *Sjögren syndrome:* Neurologic manifestations of Sjögren syndrome include seizures, movement disorders, psychiatric symptoms, aseptic meningitis, symptoms mimicking multiple sclerosis, and even a progressive dementia.

   PNS involvement (occurring in 25% of patients) includes polyneuropathy, characteristically a sensory neuropathy. Spinal cord involvement includes progressive myelopathy, transverse myelopathy, Brown–Séquard syndrome, neurogenic bladder, and spinal subarachnoid hemorrhage. Sjögren syndrome also is associated with neuromuscular disorders, including myasthenia gravis, polymyositis, and inclusion body myositis. Treatment of CNS Sjögren syndrome involves the use of steroids or cyclophosphamide. **Some patients with Sjögren syndrome** develop leptomeningeal enhancement on MRI with a progressive dementia that may respond to steroid treatment.

3. *Rheumatoid arthritis (RA):* Neurologic manifestations of RA most often occur in patients with long-standing disease and with positive rheumatoid factor. Compression or entrapment neuropathy occurs when swollen tissues compress peripheral nerves (e.g., carpal tunnel syndrome). Sensorimotor neuropathy is less common, is progressive, and can be disabling. Myelopathy also can affect patients with RA, because the cervical spine frequently is involved, and the cervical canal can become narrowed during neck flexion after atlantoaxial subluxation. Posterior circulation symptoms, including vertigo and weakness, can occur because of vertebral artery flow compromise by compression or thrombosis.

4. *Sarcoidosis:* Granulomas in the CNS can occur in extradural, subdural, leptomeningeal, and parenchymal locations, causing a wide spectrum of CNS symptoms that include:
   • Aseptic meningitis with headache, lethargy, vomiting, papilledema, and meningismus.
   • Hydrocephalus, secondary to granulomatous obstruction of cerebrospinal fluid (CSF).
   • Basilar meningitis affecting cranial nerves VII through XII and the optic nerve.
   • Granulomas in the cerebral hemispheres, which can cause progressive dementia and epileptic foci.

   Sarcoidosis, hypercalcemia, or opportunistic infections also may cause neurologic symptoms. Occasionally, patients have a hypothalamic syndrome, which may include disturbance affecting appetite, sleep, salt and water balance, and behavior. Cerebrospinal fluid (CSF) usually shows elevated protein, a mononuclear pleocytosis, and decreased glucose. Peripheral neuropathy with mononeuritis multiplex, or slowly progressive symmetric sensorimotor neuropathy also is seen. **Sarcoidosis is one of the "great masqueraders" and may affect any part of the nervous system.**

5. *Vasculitis: CNS vasculitis* may cause headache, behavioral changes, memory impairment, psychiatric symptoms, alteration in consciousness, and generalized seizures. Focal cerebral deficits with a stroke-like picture can be caused by vasculitis and should be considered, particularly in a young patient. Cranial nerve palsies also may occur. Neurologic symptoms may be the only initial manifestation of a systemic vasculitis.

   In the peripheral nervous system (PNS), mononeuritis multiplex and a distal symmetric "stocking glove" sensorimotor polyneuropathy may occur. Patients experience severe, burning dysesthetic pain in the distribution of the involved nerves. Patients may have an elevated erythrocyte sedimentation rate, CSF protein, and lymphocytic pleocytosis in the CSF during active disease. Magnetic resonance imaging (MRI) demonstrates small areas of cerebral infarction. However, a brain, leptomeningeal, or peripheral nerve biopsy specimen is often necessary to make a definitive diagnosis of CNS or PNS vasculitis. Treatment involves removing possible inciting antigens such as medications, infectious agents, or environmental toxins. Immunosuppressive therapy with corticosteroids and cytotoxic drugs (especially cyclophosphamide) can be helpful.

OTHER DISORDERS

1. *PRES: Posterior reversible encephalopathy syndrome* has been described in patients with several acute systemic illnesses. Symptoms include headache, altered mental function, seizures, and a striking loss of vision; accompanied by reversible white matter changes on MRI. Treatment of hypertension or removal of offending medications such as cyclosporine may hasten recovery. Occasionally, such patients show evidence of vasospasm, complicating treatment strategies.

2. *Organ transplantation* is commonly accompanied by neurologic disorders. These complications relate to the operation, immunosuppressive medications, infections, graft versus host, other immunologic reactions, and secondary effects of organ failure.

3. *Critical illness* is accompanied by many neurologic problems. Critical illness polyneuropathy is a syndrome in patients with long-term, complicated intensive care unit (ICU) stays, who develop a severe neuropathy that causes quadriparesis, and may affect respiratory muscles. The specific etiology is unknown, but sepsis is implicated in its pathogenesis. Tight glucose control in the ICU appears to reduce the incidence and severity of critical illness polyneuropathy. Seizures, hypoxic-ischemic disease, stroke, and metabolic encephalopathy are common in the ICU. A prolonged neuromuscular paralysis sometimes is seen after the use of paralyzing agents; particularly in the presence of renal failure. Similarly, a severe myopathy sometimes is seen in the ICU after intravenous steroid therapy.

Suggested Readings

Als-Nielsen B, Gluud LL, Gluud C. Nonabsorbable disaccharides for hepatic encephalopathy. *Cochrane Database Syst Rev.* 2004;2:CD003044.

Ballerini L, Cifarelli A, Ammirati A, et al. Patent foramen ovale and cryptogenic stroke. A critical review. *J Cardiovasc Med (Hagerstown).* 2007;8:34–38.

Bronster DJ, Emre S, Boccagni P, et al. Central nervous system complications in liver transplant recipients—incidence, timing, and long-term follow-up. *Clin Transplant.* 2000;14:1–7.

Chong JY, Rowland LP, Utiger RD. Hashimoto encephalopathy: syndrome or myth? *Arch Neurol.* 2003;60:164–171.

Covarrubias DJ, Luetmer PH, Campeau NG. Posterior reversible encephalopathy syndrome: prognostic utility of quantitative diffusion-weighted MR images. *AJNR.* 2002;23:1038–1048.

Gerard A, Sarrot-Reynauld F, Liozon E, et al. Neurologic presentation of Whipple disease: report of 12 cases and review of the literature. *Medicine (Baltimore).* 2002;81:443–457.

Ghezzi A, Zaffaroni M. Neurological manifestations of gastrointestinal disorders, with particular reference to the differential diagnosis of multiple sclerosis. *Neurol Sci.* 2001;22(suppl 2): S117–S122.

Hypothermia after Cardiac Arrest Study Group. Mild therapeutic hypothermia to improve the neurologic outcome after cardiac arrest. *NEJM.* 2002;346:549–556.

Juhasz-Pocsine K, Rudnicki SA, Archer RL, et al. Neurologic complications of gastric bypass surgery for morbid obesity. *Neurology.* 2007;68:1843–1850.

Kumar S, Fowler M, Gonzalez-Toledo E, et al. Central pontine myelinolysis, an update. *Neurol Res.* 2006;28:360–366.

Kwan JY. Paraproteinemic neuropathy. *Neurol Clin.* 2007;25: 47–69.

Muscal E, Brey RL. Neurological manifestations of the antiphospholipid syndrome: risk assessments and evidence-based medicine. *Int J Clin Pract.* 2007;61:1561–1568.

Scheid R, Teich N. Neurologic manifestations of ulcerative colitis. *Eur J Neurol.* 2007;14:483–493.

Schilsky ML. Wilson disease: new insights into pathogenesis, diagnosis, and future therapy. *Curr Gastroenterol Rep.* 2005;7:26–31.

Scott TF, Yandora K, Valeri A, et al. Aggressive therapy for neurosarcoidosis: long-term follow-up of 48 treated patients. *Arch Neurol.* 2007;64:691–696.

Shawcross D, Jalan R. Dispelling myths in the treatment of hepatic encephalopathy. *Lancet*. 2005;365:431–433.

Zivković SJ. Neuroimaging and neurologic complications after organ transplantation. *Neuroimaging*. 2007;17:110–123.

29 Treatment of Pain in Neurologic Disease

A working understanding of pain and its treatment is important in the management of many patients with neurologic disease. Consider the following points:

1. Pain is a subjective symptom. There are no physical findings that quantify or exclude the presence of pain. Assume that the patient has pain, and then approach management.
2. An adequate pain assessment includes documentation of pain location, intensity, quality, onset, duration, variation, what makes it worse, what makes it better, effects of pain on function and lifestyle, and the development of a pain plan.
3. It is important to consider disease factors that may cause pain, and evaluate the patient appropriately for pain-causing disorders that can be corrected (e.g., tumor causing pain, compressive nerve root lesion).
4. Pain can be quantified by the patient. Numerous studies have shown that a visual analog scale, in which the patient bisects a line that goes from "no pain" to "maximal pain," is the best method of quantifying pain. It is simple and provides the physician with a "semi-objective" measure of whether pain is improving or worsening.
5. Patients with chronic pain often develop depression, and are misunderstood by physicians, or shunned as "difficult" patients. In addition, there may be workers' compensation or litigation issues that complicate the doctor–patient relationship. The physician may develop "compassion fatigue" when dealing with a chronically disabled patient in pain. Chronic pain is often best managed in a center with comprehensive services.

TREATMENT OF PAIN

It is best to use a "stepped" approach in pain management.

1. Begin with simple analgesics such as acetaminophen, aspirin, and nonsteroidal medications.

2. Addition of a tricyclic antidepressant may be useful in chronic pain, neuropathic pain, and headache, and in depressed patients with pain. Gradual titration of the medication dose usually works best. Amitriptyline, imipramine, and nortriptyline are commonly used, and have been shown to have efficacy in neuropathic pain. Selective serotonin reuptake inhibitors are less effective in pain management. Venlafaxine and nefazodone are antidepressants with potential efficacy in pain management.

3. Antiepileptic medication also may be used in chronic pain management, particularly when pain is neuropathic. Phenytoin, carbamazepine, valproic acid, and gabapentin each can be of benefit. Gabapentin is particularly useful in trigeminal neuralgia, and in painful peripheral neuropathy. Gabapentin has minimal interaction with other medications. Pre-gabalin is FDA approved for painful diabetic neuropathy and has also been used for other neuropathic pain syndromes. Both gabapentin and pre-gabalin are renally excreted and dose adjustments need to be made for renal dysfunction. Other newer antiepileptic medications such as lamotrigine, topiramate, and levetiracetam also are used for this indication.

4. Steroids may be used in certain situations; particularly for short-term therapy in patients with cancer.

5. Low-potency narcotic medication may be useful (e.g., codeine in combination with aspirin, acetaminophen, or propoxyphene).

6. Higher-potency narcotic medications are used when there is cancer-related pain, for short-term acute severe pain, or in a controlled program in chronic neuropathic pain. Patients who have pain and are not "drug seeking" are at low risk of addiction with such medications. The patient plays an important role in therapy and must be educated by the physician. Thus, there is no "right" dose for pain control, and the dose must be titrated with the patient's help to be most effective. Useful medications include oxycodone, morphine in various preparations, and transdermal fentanyl. In acute postoperative pain, patient-controlled analgesia with an intravenous pump is effective. Occasionally, methadone may be beneficial. It is important to have a contract for care for the use of chronic narcotics that sets out the appropriate use of long-term narcotics, the responsibilities of the patient, and rules for conduct that the patient must follow to continue medication use (e.g., not "losing prescriptions," not changing dose without physician approval).

7. Providing pain medications before they are needed (i.e., a regular dosing) is better than on a demand basis. By providing

the pain medication regularly, the total dose required may be lower, and patient discomfort will be lessened while waiting for the next dose to take effect.

8. Topical therapies may be useful in focal pain syndromes. Capsaicin cream may be helpful with a painful joint or in distal foot pain from neuropathy. Lidocaine 5% patches may be useful, particularly for focal pain syndromes such as post-herpetic neuralgia. These patches should be used in a "12 hours on, 12 hours off protocol" to limit side effects.

9. Nonpharmacologic approaches to pain management may be helpful. These include physical measures such as warm or cold compresses, transcutaneous electrical nerve stimulators, massage therapy, chiropractic manipulation, and acupuncture; behavioral therapy such as biofeedback and relaxation therapy; and exercise and stretching programs.

10. *Surgical approaches* are used in refractory pain disorders. Surgical approaches are limited by cost and morbidity. The most common procedures include implanted pumps for baclofen, morphine for spasticity and spinal cord pain, spinal cord stimulators for refractory low back pain syndromes, thalamic stimulators for central pain syndromes, and dorsal root entry zone lesions for focal root and refractory trigeminal neuralgia.

NOTES ON BACK PAIN

Back pain is one of the most common problems that physicians see. Many neurologists are called upon to assist in the diagnosis and treatment of back pain. The following are a few factors to consider when presented with such patients:

1. Most acute back pain will resolve spontaneously whatever treatment course is prescribed or self-prescribed. There is no evidence that bed rest of any kind is beneficial.

2. Patients with progressive pain, systemic symptoms, or focal neurologic symptoms or signs, warrant early investigations. Otherwise conservative management for the first few weeks is reasonable.

3. The back examination is of limited use in the differential diagnosis of back pain. However, it makes the patient more comfortable if the back is assessed by the physician.

4. Chiropractic manipulation has been shown to be as effective as medical care for acute low back pain.

5. Physical therapy and exercise are beneficial.

6. Surgical therapy of low back pain without focal neurologic findings is usually avoided unless there are no other options, and is rarely curative.

7. The judicious use of nonsteroidals and/or muscle relaxants may be helpful, but habit-forming medication should be avoided in this patient population. Various injection techniques may be helpful in selected patients.

8. Disability is a common issue in chronic back pain, and should be addressed formally by a physiatrist or occupational specialist if possible.

Suggested Readings

Attal N, Cruccu G, Haanpaa M, et al. EFNS Task Force. EFNS guidelines on pharmacological treatment of neuropathic pain. *Eur J Neurol.* 2006;13:1153–1169.

Boswell MV, Trescot AM, Datta S, et al. Interventional techniques: evidence-based practice guidelines in the management of chronic spinal pain. *Pain Phys.* 2007;10:7–111.

Bradley LA, McKendree-Smith NL. Central nervous system mechanisms of pain in fibromyalgia and other musculoskeletal disorders: behavioral and psychologic treatment approaches. *Curr Opin Rheumatol.* 2002;14:45–51.

Eisenberg E, McNicol E, Carr DB. Opioids for neuropathic pain. *Cochrane Database Syst Rev.* 2006;3:CD006146.

Lumbar Puncture and Cerebrospinal Fluid

INDICATIONS

1. When central nervous system (CNS) infection (meningitis, encephalitis) is suspected, one must examine the cerebrospinal fluid (CSF). However, there is an exception: lumbar puncture (LP) should not be performed if one suspects brain abscess or another significant space-occupying mass lesion.

2. An LP is performed to diagnose subarachnoid hemorrhage when that diagnosis is strongly suspected, and the computed tomography (CT) scan result is negative.

3. An LP is done when cerebrospinal fluid (CSF) chemistries may have diagnostic value (e.g., gamma globulin and oligoclonal banding in multiple sclerosis).

4. LP is needed for the study of CSF *pressure:*
   - To check for increased pressure in suspected pseudotumor cerebri.
   - To check for low pressure in spontaneous intracranial hypotension headache.
   - In normal pressure hydrocephalus, when removal of CSF may improve gait and mentation.

5. LP is done for cytology, when carcinomatous or lymphomatous meningitis is suspected. Remember to take large volumes for cytology. First tap results are often negative, and a second or third tap may be required to demonstrate abnormal cells.

6. *Therapeutically,* an LP may be done to inject methotrexate or ara-c for central nervous system (CNS) leukemia, or amphotericin B for fungal meningitis, or to remove fluid as treatment for benign increased intracranial pressure.

CONTRAINDICATIONS

Contraindications to LP include the following:

1. Infection at the site of the LP.
2. Severe thrombocytopenia or uncorrected bleeding disorder.

3. When a cerebral *mass lesion* (brain abscess, brain tumor, etc.) is suspected, particularly in a patient with lateralized neurologic signs or a possible mass in the posterior fossa.

4. *Intracranial hemorrhage.* This condition is best diagnosed by CT scan. In these instances, a CT scan, or magnetic resonance imaging (MRI) for definition of the hemorrhage, and a search for a mass lesion should be done before the LP.

5. *Spinal block.* This is a relative contraindication to a lumbar puncture (LP); a CT scan or MRI should be done before considering an LP.

6. *Presence of papilledema* (a check of the fundi must precede each LP) without radiologic examination. An LP ultimately may be done in a patient with papilledema (e.g., in pseudotumor or if CSF examination is crucial), but only after neurologic or neurosurgical consultation.

7. *In the presence of spinal epidural abscess.* Performing an LP in this setting may spread infection to the CSF.

8. Clopidogrel may be a contraindication to LP, due to increased risk of epidural bleeding. Similarly anticoagulants are a contraindication to LP.

COMPLICATIONS

Post–lumbar puncture (LP) headache occurs in 10% to 30% of patients. It is characteristically exacerbated by sitting or standing, and it is relieved by lying flat. It is seen within the first 1 to 3 days after the LP; it usually lasts 2 to 5 days, although it may persist for weeks. Treatment consists of bed rest and fluids. The mechanism of the headache is believed to be continued CSF leakage through the dural hole at the site of the LP, with subsequent intracranial traction on the meninges. Caffeinated beverages, ergot preparations, and theophylline may be helpful in this headache. Severe leaks can be treated by the placement of a blood patch by an anesthesiologist or neurosurgeon. Post-LP headache may be minimized by using a small-gauge needle (22) (type A recommendation), inserting the needle parallel to the dural fibers so they are spread apart rather than torn, and having the patient turn prone before removing the needle. The diagnostic lumbar puncture data for noncutting needles versus cutting needles are inconclusive. Having the patient lie in bed after LP does not appear to reduce the incidence of post-LP headache, and no longer is recommended. Patients with migraine are particularly prone to post-LP headaches.

When there is an unexpected *increased opening pressure* (it must stay elevated after the patient has relaxed with legs extended, and a few minutes have elapsed from the onset of the LP), remove minimal fluid needed for studies. One may leave the needle in with the stopcock closed to prevent further leakage.

Neurologic or neurosurgical consultation should be obtained, the use of mannitol or steroids should be considered, and the patient should be watched carefully over the ensuing hours for signs of deterioration. Patients with meningitis may have markedly elevated pressures, but these pressures are not as severe a risk as increased intracranial pressure secondary to a focal lesion. Remember, hypercarbia, water intoxication, and hypertensive encephalopathy are remediable causes of increased intracranial pressure. When the intracranial pressure is increased, and there is neurologic deterioration immediately or during the hours after the LP, treatment with osmotic dehydrating agents and steroids is indicated (see Chapter 31). In cryptococcal meningitis, acutely elevated CSF pressures may lead to blindness from optic nerve pressure, even when CT scan is normal. Treatment with continuous lumbar or ventricular drainage, in combination with antibiotics, is usually effective.

If the patient has a partial or almost complete *spinal block* secondary to compression of the cord (e.g., by tumor), CSF removal may cause rapid worsening of the block. Signs of block include abnormal manometric findings and xanthochromic fluid (yellow, thick CSF due to increased protein) under low pressure (see Chapter 9 for treatment).

METHOD

The puncture is carried out in the midline between the L4 to L5, or L5 to S1 interspaces located by the level of the iliac crest.

1. Insert the bevel of the needle parallel to the long axis of the spine.
2. Note the opening and closing pressures, and the amount of fluid removed.
3. Coughing or abdominal pressure causes delayed venous return around the cord and should increase CSF flow and pressure. These maneuvers show that the needle is in place, but they do not test for spinal subarachnoid block. To do this, increase the jugular pressure (with hand pressure or a blood pressure cuff around the neck) and measure the rise and fall of CSF pressure. Manometric studies are not done routinely and are never

performed if the baseline pressure is elevated, or an intracranial lesion is suspected.

4. *Proper positioning* of the patient is crucial for successful LP. The patient should be placed in the fetal position with the patient's back at right angles to the bed. Insert the needle under the skin (after local anesthesia), and then decide on the angle of entry. Make sure the needle is strictly perpendicular to the patient's waist and angled toward the umbilicus. If the LP is impossible in the fetal position, have the patient sit up and lean forward over the bedside table, grasping a pillow; try again in the sitting position (it is easier to gauge the midline).

When an LP is impossible because of bony anomalies or local infection, and CSF examination is crucial, one should arrange for a lumbar puncture under fluoroscopy. Rarely, cisternal or cervical (C1–C2) punctures under fluoroscopy may be beneficial (occasionally in malignant leptomeningeal disease).

EXAMINATION OF THE CEREBROSPINAL FLUID

1. If red blood cells (RBCs) are present, count them in the first and fourth tubes. In subarachnoid or intracranial bleeding, the amount of blood remains constant in each tube and the blood does not clot. Decreasing numbers of cells suggest a traumatic tap. After centrifugation, the CSF from a traumatic tap will be clear, whereas with true CNS bleeding, the supernatant is xanthochromic if the bleeding occurred at least 2 to 4 hours previously.

2. Check to see if the CSF is *clear* by comparing it with water. A CSF protein level greater than 100 mg/dL usually causes the spinal fluid to look faintly yellow. Approximately 200 to 300 white blood cells (WBCs) are needed to cause CSF cloudiness. Dark CSF may be seen with metastatic melanoma, and jaundice with hyperbilirubinemia; subdural hematoma may produce xanthochromia.

3. Always examine the CSF for *cells*. Normally, there should be no polymorphonuclear neutrophils (PMNs) and no more than 5 mononuclear cells. When looking for tumor cells, or if the nature of the WBCs in the CSF is questioned, a cytologic examination is indicated. When bacterial or tuberculous infection is suspected, perform a Gram stain and an acid-fast stain on the centrifuged sediment. When fungal disease is a possibility, do an India ink preparation.

4. When there are RBCs in the CSF and the patient has a normal complete blood count, expect approximately 1 WBC for every

700 RBCs (make further corrections for anemia). In addition, every 700 RBCs increase the protein by approximately 1 mg/dL.
5. Flow cytometry may increase the identification of neoplastic cells in patients with leptomeningeal carcinomatosis or lymphomatosis. Discuss storage media and transmission with the laboratory to optimize the analysis of the spinal fluid.

INTERPRETATION

Glucose

Increased glucose levels are usually insignificant, merely reflecting systemic hyperglycemia. With changing blood glucose, CSF glucose lags blood glucose by approximately 1 hour, and the level is approximately two-thirds that of blood glucose. With systemic hyperglycemia, a concomitant blood glucose determination is needed to demonstrate a relatively decreased CSF glucose (e.g., suggesting infection) that may otherwise be considered normal.

Decreased glucose levels are seen in bacterial, tuberculous, and fungal meningitis, and sometimes with meningeal involvement by neoplasm, or a nontuberculous granulomatous process, such as sarcoidosis. Although characteristically normal in viral infections, the CSF glucose level has been reported to be low with certain CNS viral infections (herpes, mumps, lymphocytic choriomeningitis).

Protein

Protein levels are increased in many neurologic diseases and usually reflect an abnormality in the blood–brain barrier. Elevated levels are seen in processes affecting nerve roots in peripheral neuropathy. Normal CSF protein is less than 45 mg/dL. Common processes producing increased CSF protein are as follows:

1. *Diabetes* frequently causes protein elevations (up to 150 mg/dL, or even higher when significant peripheral neuropathy is present).
2. *Spinal cord tumors* also increase protein levels, often to extremely high levels (e.g., 750–1,000 mg/dL), especially when a block is present.
3. *Multiple sclerosis* may cause protein elevation in some patients, but the elevation is usually mild. Protein levels greater than 80 mg/dL in a patient with multiple sclerosis make the diagnosis suspect.

4. *Acute purulent meningitis* invariably elevates the protein level regardless of the cause, as do subacute and chronic granulomatous meningitis. Viral infections of the CNS are associated with normal protein levels, or mild increases in protein initially with an increase later, which serves as a clue to the diagnosis. Carcinomatous meningitis causes significant elevation of CSF protein.

5. *Infectious polyneuritis* (Guillain–Barré syndrome) characteristically causes increased protein levels. The protein is frequently normal during the first few days of the illness, but increases after 1 week.

6. *Syphilis* produces increased protein levels in the meningovascular form and general paresis; the CSF may be normal in long-standing tabes.

7. Mild to moderate elevations may be seen in myxedema, uremia, connective tissue disorders, and Cushing disease.

Gamma Globulin

The measurement of gamma globulin is used most frequently to support the diagnosis of multiple sclerosis. Normally, gamma globulin represents 13% to 15% or less of total protein. (If total protein values are less than 20 mg/100 mL, the percentage of gamma globulin may be unreliable.) Gamma globulin is elevated in multiple sclerosis, subacute sclerosing panencephalitis, Lyme disease, general paresis, herpes encephalitis, myxedema, some cases of carcinomatous cerebellar degeneration, and some connective tissue diseases (e.g., lupus). Measurement of immunoglobulin G (IgG), albumin ratio (normally less than 0.18), measurement of IgG synthesis rate, or detection of oligoclonal bands provides similar information.

Oligoclonal bands are a marker of the production of a few clones of antibodies in the CSF (oligo = few). It is a measure of immunologic activity in the CNS compartment.

PLEOCYTOSIS

PMNs in the CSF suggest a bacterial infection, and lymphocytes suggest a viral or chronic inflammatory process (although PMNs sometimes are seen at the onset of a viral infection). WBCs may be seen after subarachnoid hemorrhage, thrombosis, and at times, with infectious mononucleosis. Eosinophils suggest a parasitic infection, chemical meningitis, or dye reaction. Remember, many organic diseases of the central nervous system produce a mild pleocytosis. A thorough bacteriologic investigation must be carried out in all instances, although cells do not always represent infection. Carcinomatous meningitis tends to be accompanied by fewer than 100 cells in the cerebrospinal fluid (more than 100 cells suggest an infectious process). T-cell and B-cell markers should be checked, if the WBC count in the CSF is elevated and lymphomatous meningitis is suspected. The initial tap may be negative for tumor cells. The yield is increased on repeated cytological examinations.

Note: If at CSF analysis the cell count, protein, and glucose are normal, it is highly unlikely that additional studies on the spinal fluid will be useful (unless it is a special consideration such as oligoclonal band determination in suspected multiple sclerosis).

CEREBROSPINAL FLUID PRESSURE

The *CSF pressure* is normally less than 200 mm H_2O with the patient lying down (or at the level of the foramen magnum in the sitting position). It is not affected by changes in systemic blood pressure, but is exquisitely sensitive to changes in blood CO_2 (hyperventilation decreases intracranial pressure) and venous pressure.

1. Elevated pressures are seen in acute bacterial, fungal, and viral meningitis and meningoencephalitis.
2. Pressure elevation is frequent with tumors, or other intracerebral mass lesions (e.g., abscess), although pressure may be normal despite a large tumor.
3. Pressure usually is elevated in intracerebral bleeding, and in subarachnoid hemorrhage.
4. It is interesting that the pressure and protein may be increased, and there may be papilledema with polyneuritis or spinal tumor.
5. Unexplained elevated pressures may be caused by congestive heart failure, chronic obstructive pulmonary disease, hypercapnia, jugular venous obstruction, or pericardial effusion.
6. Pseudotumor cerebri (benign increased intracranial pressure) refers to increased pressure; as high as 400 to 600 mm H_2O with papilledema, not associated with a mass lesion, or hydrocephalus, and with an otherwise normal CSF. Causes include withdrawal from steroids, pregnancy and menarche, excess vitamin A, hyperparathyroidism, tetracycline or phenothiazine administration, and venous sinus occlusion. Patients with pseudotumor are frequently obese. The cause of pseudotumor

cerebri is unknown. One must first rule out tumor and hydrocephalus (usually with CT scan or MRI), and then establish the diagnosis with a lumbar puncture. LPs alone are sometimes sufficient to decrease CSF pressure and reverse the process. Acetazolamide may be given to decrease CSF production, and then steroids are administered if necessary. Transient visual disturbances, such as blurring and dimming, are common in pseudotumor. More severe visual difficulties, such as field defects and actual loss of vision, also can occur and warrant vigorous treatment of the increased pressure; including lumboperitoneal shunts in protracted cases. Optic nerve sheath fenestration may prevent blindness in some cases. Frequent monitoring of visual fields and of the optic nerve is warranted.

7. Patients may develop *spontaneous intracranial hypotension headache*. This is a positional headache, worse with sitting and standing, similar to a post-LP headache but without an apparent cause. On LP, there is no pleocytosis but there is a low CSF pressure. MRI scanning with gadolinium shows diffuse meningeal enhancement, and there is often downward sagging of the brainstem on sagittal views. This disorder may be treated with fluids, steroids, and sometimes a blood patch. Nuclear medicine cisternography may show a dural tear in some cases.

Suggested Readings

Armon C, Evans RW. Addendum to assessment: prevention of post-lumbar puncture headaches: report of the Therapeutics and Technology Assessment Subcommittee of the American Academy of Neurology. *Neurology*. 2005;65:510–512.

Burgett RA, Purvin VA, Kawasaki A. Lumboperitoneal shunting for pseudotumor cerebri. *Neurology*. 1997;49:734–739.

Evans RW. Complications of lumbar puncture. *Neurol Clin*. 1998;16:83–105.

Holdgate A, Cuthbert K. Perils and pitfalls of lumbar puncture in the emergency department. *Emerg Med*. 2001;13:351–358.

Radharkrishnan K, Ahlskog JE, Garrity JA, et al. Idiopathic intracranial hypertension. *Mayo Clin Proc*. 1994;69:169–180.

Schievink WI. Spontaneous spinal cerebrospinal fluid leaks and intracranial hypotension. *JAMA*. 2006;295:2286–2296.

31 Increased Intracranial Pressure

CASE

A 47-year-old man comes to the emergency room after one week of high fever and headache. Today he became progressively weaker on his right side and now cannot speak. As you examine him he vomits, becomes unresponsive, and begins to extend his arms and legs stiffly. His left pupil is dilated and sluggishly reactive. His stat CT scan shows a mass lesion in the left hemisphere with massive edema and left to right shift.

Diagnosis

Cerebral abscess with lateral herniation syndrome.

Increased intracranial pressure may be secondary to a focal mass lesion or more diffuse processes. *Signs* and *symptoms* include headache, nausea and vomiting, lethargy, diplopia (usually secondary to a sixth-nerve palsy), transient visual obscurations, and papilledema. As intracranial pressure continues to increase, there may be bradycardia (50 to 60 beats/min), elevation of blood pressure, increase in systolic pressure associated with lowering or slight elevation of diastolic pressure, and a slowing of the respiratory rate (Cushing reflex).

Papilledema, when present, is a useful sign. The presence of venous pulsations suggests a normal cerebrospinal fluid (CSF) pressure and makes it unlikely that intracranial pressure is present. On funduscopic examination, venous pulsations are best visualized where the vein turns and emerges from the optic nerve head.

HERNIATION SYNDROMES

There are three clinical syndromes of transtentorial herniation. Two represent loss of neurologic function that begins in the cerebral hemispheres and progresses to involve upper and then lower brainstem, which is fatal if untreated. The third and most uncommon consists of upward herniation of posterior fossa structures; it also can be fatal.

Lateral (Uncal) Syndrome of Herniation

1. A unilaterally dilated pupil is the first sign secondary to a mass in the middle fossa. Traditionally, it was taught that this is the result of compression of the third nerve against the incisura. However, magnetic resonance imaging (MRI) studies have shown that third-nerve paresis is more commonly caused by distortion of the midbrain rather than direct third nerve compression. There is a close correlation between the degree of lateral displacement and the alteration of consciousness. A contralateral hemiplegia usually is present. Respiration and consciousness usually are unimpaired. Sometimes the ipsilateral pupil is small, rather than large, and rarely the contralateral pupil dilates before the ipsilateral one.

2. Progressive pressure increase leads to increasing stupor, a more complete third-nerve palsy, and sometimes an ipsilateral hemiplegia with bilateral Babinski responses. The ipsilateral hemiparesis is secondary to tentorial pressure against the opposite cerebral peduncle (Kernohan notch). Respiration may be normal or of the central neurogenic hyperventilation pattern. There is often decerebrate posturing (arms extended at the side with inward turning, spontaneously or when a noxious stimulus is applied). Decorticate posturing (arms flexed at the elbow "pointing" to the cortex) is not usually seen with the uncal syndrome.

Central Syndrome of Herniation

Pressure is exerted centrally on the diencephalon, rather than laterally as occurs in the lateral or uncal syndrome. The first sign is a change in alertness or behavior. Respiration is usually normal and contains frequent sighs or yawns. There may be Cheyne–Stokes respirations. Brainstem function is intact, although pupils are small but reactive to light, and there may be roving eye movements. Bilateral hyperreflexia and Babinski responses and rigidity of the extremities are usual. With progression, there is decorticate posturing and coma.

Posterior Fossa Herniation Syndrome

1. Posterior fossa lesions may cause damage by direct compression of the brainstem and by upward herniation through the

tentorial hiatus. Upward herniation from the posterior fossa obliterates the ambient cisterns and aqueduct, causing hydrocephalus with obtundation or coma.

2. Midbrain compression produces an upward gaze deficit, whereas involvement of pontine pathways may cause sixth-nerve palsies, ocular bobbing, and other oculomotor signs. In addition, anisocoria (asymmetric pupils) may progress to mid-position fixed pupils. *Ocular bobbing* refers to a sudden conjugate downward deviation of the eyes, followed by a slow, upward drift. It often is seen in pontine hemorrhage with coma and quadriparesis. These syndromes can develop over hours or minutes, depending on the pathologic process.

AGENTS USED IN TREATING INTRACRANIAL PRESSURE

Hyperventilation

Hyperventilation may be used in acute situations (e.g., head trauma) and often is used during neurosurgical procedures. Lowering the pCO_2 to 25 to 30 mm Hg causes vasoconstriction, reduced cerebral blood flow, an immediate reduction in intracerebral blood volume, and thus a decrease of intracranial pressure. Decreasing pCO_2 to less than 25 mm Hg may be harmful because it reduces cerebral blood flow. Hyperventilation is only of transient benefit.

■ Mannitol

Mannitol, an osmotic dehydrating agent, may be used. A common adult dose is 25 to 50 g initially followed by 12.5 to 25 g every 6 hours, depending on serum osmolarity. Onset of action is 15 to 30 minutes. It draws intracerebral water into the intravascular space because of its hypertonicity and, for the same reason, induces diuresis. It is usually not given for more than 24 to 48 hours and is used in acute situations to "buy time" (e.g., after head trauma, deterioration from an expanding intracranial process), often before neurosurgical intervention.

Urea is similar to mannitol in its use, mode of action, and dose. These agents must be given with caution to patients with renal and cardiac disease. There may be "rebound" after their use (viz., return of water intracerebrally) because small amounts cross the blood–brain barrier. Lower doses of mannitol (250 mg/kg) reduce the rebound brain edema sometimes seen with mannitol.

Diuretics such as furosemide often are given as a supplement to mannitol. An osmolarity of approximately 300 to 310 mOsm/L appears to be optimal. Electrolytes and osmolarity should be checked as clinically indicated, usually every 12 hours in an acute situation.

■ Steroids

Steroids (e.g., dexamethasone) are used acutely and chronically (10 mg IV as initial bolus, then 4 to 6 mg IV intramuscularly or orally every 4 to 6 hours). The onset of action is approximately 12 hours. Dexamethasone is given in acute situations and may become the mainstay of treatment after 12 to 24 hours. Dexamethasone is used to treat the vasogenic edema associated with brain tumor and abscess, after some neurosurgical procedures, and often concomitantly with radiation therapy to the brain. The mechanism of steroid action in these situations is poorly understood. Patients receiving steroids for more than a few hours usually receive cimetidine, ranitidine, or oral antacids. Steroids are probably not beneficial in treating adults with trauma-induced cerebral edema or for cytotoxic edema associated with hypoxia, cerebral infarcts, or cerebral hemorrhage.

■ Hypertonic Saline

Recent studies in the ICU setting, particularly in patients on ventilators with continuous intracranial pressure monitoring, have shown that intermittent dosing with hypertonic saline (varied concentrations) effectively reduced intracranial pressure in a variety of conditions. The use of this agent should be limited to patients where close monitoring, particularly of intracranial pressures, is available.

Ventricular Drainage

Ventricular puncture and drainage may be done by a neurosurgeon when acute hydrocephalus occurs and mechanical release of increased intracranial pressure is needed. Ventricular puncture and placement of an intraventricular catheter may be done in the emergency room or in the intensive care unit. Lumbar drainage may be useful in some meningitides such as cryptococcal meningitis because an acute block of CSF flow requires artificial means to remove CSF. If untreated, blindness and coma may occur as a result of a decreased cerebral perfusion pressure (mean arterial pressure minus intracranial pressure).

■ Barbiturates

A controversial contribution to intracranial pressure control is the use of barbiturates. They usually are used when other attempts to decrease intracranial pressure have failed and should be used only in conjunction with an intraventricular pressure monitor in an intensive care unit. Pentobarbital is the most widely used agent. Its mechanism of action in reducing intracranial pressure is unknown.

Note: Metabolic factors such as hypoxia, hypercarbia, and hyperthermia can increase intracranial pressure. Twisted neck positions leading to kinking of the jugular veins and high mean airway pressures also can increase intracranial pressure. Hyperthermia invariably increases intracranial pressure and should be managed aggressively.

Suggested Readings

Brazis PW, Lee AG. Elevated intracranial pressure and pseudotumor cerebri. *Curr Opin Opthalmol.* 1998;9:27–32.

McDonald C, Carter BS. Medical management of increased intracranial pressure after spontaneous intracerebral hemorrhage. *Neurosurg Clin North Am.* 2002;13:335–338.

Roberts I, Schierhout G, Wakai A. Mannitol for acute traumatic brain injury. *Cochrane Database Syst Rev.* 2003;2:CD001049.

Schwarz S, Georgiadis D, Aschoff A, et al. Effects of hypertonic (10%) saline in patients with raised intracranial pressure after stroke. *Stroke.* 2002;33:136–140.

Traumatic Brain Injury

Damage to the brain after trauma may be caused by direct injury from bone fragments or penetrating missiles; impact of brain against the base of the skull; shearing forces causing axonal injury within the white matter; or secondary phenomena such as hematomas, edema, and anoxic injury caused by respiratory difficulty. Rapid assessment and resuscitation are crucial in reducing secondary damage and preserving the potential for recovery. Head injury is a major cause of death and disability at all ages, particularly in people younger than age 25 years.

Head injury is a dynamic process. The most important parameters to monitor are the patient's level of consciousness and mental status. Following are important guidelines in dealing with the patient with head trauma.

1. In *severe head trauma*, control of airway and intravenous line placement are first priorities. One should assume that the patient has a fractured cervical spine and avoid turning the head; obtain cervical spine films in addition to skull films. Search for accompanying traumatic injury to abdominal and thoracic organs. If a patient has head injury and shock, assume that they are unrelated. Most patients are cared for in major trauma centers that use protocols for initial evaluation and resuscitation. Systematic approaches to trauma management help to avoid overlooking injuries that may not be initially apparent.

2. In obtaining the patient's *history*, establish the mode of injury and whether there was an associated anoxic period. Were there other factors such as drug and alcohol ingestion, exposure and hypothermia, or other medical problems? Patients who "talk and then deteriorate" are at high risk of harboring an intracranial hematoma and may require immediate neurosurgical intervention.

3. All patients with head trauma require *neurologic examination*, which must include (i) careful documentation of the patient's level of consciousness and ability to carry out mental tasks, (ii) a careful look at the tympanic membranes for evidence of basilar skull fracture (blood or cerebrospinal fluid), (iii) scalp examination for evidence of localized areas of trauma,

(iv) precise recording of pupillary size and reaction, and (v) a check for hemiparesis and presence or absence of upgoing toes. The Glasgow Coma Scale, a simple and reproducible scale that allows comparison of the patient's state at different times, also should be done as part of the examination (Table 32.1).

4. *Concussion* is defined as an immediate and transient loss of consciousness or other neurological function after head injury. There may be amnesia for events before (retrograde) or after (anterograde) the amnesia.

5. *Observation in the hospital* for 24 to 48 hours and *neurosurgical consultation* are appropriate for a patient with any focal abnormalities on neurological examination, unconsciousness, abnormal mental status, skull fracture, intracranial abnormalities on computed tomography (CT), or head trauma that is thought to be significant despite a normal examination. The decision to hospitalize or send a patient home who has not been unconscious and who has a normal neurologic examination may be made after careful consideration of the severity of trauma and of who will look after and monitor the patient at home.

6. Patients who return to an emergency room within 48 hours of transfer to the community with any persistent complaint

■ TABLE 32.1. Glasgow Coma Scale

Category	Score
Eyes Open	
Never	1
To pain	2
To verbal stimuli	3
Spontaneously	4
Best Verbal Response	
None	1
Incomprehensible	2
Inappropriate words	3
Disoriented, conversing	4
Oriented, conversing	5
Best Motor Response	
None	1
Extension	2
Flexion abnormal	3
Flexion withdrawal	4
Localizing pain	5
Obeys commands	6
Total Maximum Score	15

relating to the initial head injury should be seen by or discussed with a senior clinician experienced in head injuries, and considered for a CT scan (grade B recommendation).

7. One of the most feared complications of head injury is the development of an acute *subdural or epidural hematoma*, which then may cause herniation (see Chapter 31) and fatal brainstem compression. Clinically, this process manifests itself as headache; decreased level of consciousness; and, late in the course, a dilated pupil that is usually on the side of the hematoma, secondary to pressure on the third nerve. *Epidural hematoma* most commonly represents arterial bleeding secondary to tearing the middle meningeal artery on the undersurface of the temporal bone. The patient may deteriorate after the trauma or experience a "lucid interval" only to deteriorate later. Most patients will have a fracture over the groove of the middle meningeal artery. *Subdural hematoma* is secondary to venous or arterial bleeding and also has the potential for brainstem compression. Subdural and epidural hematomas are diagnosed by CT scan or magnetic resonance imaging (MRI). *Chronic subdural hematomas* can present days or weeks after trauma, often in the elderly, and may cause slow behavioral changes, gait disturbances, headache, and incontinence.

8. Aside from the asymptomatic patient with no or very brief loss of consciousness, all patients should undergo CT scanning. Skull radiographs are not useful in most head injuries and will miss many significant intracranial abnormalities. CT scanning is helpful in assessing the type and severity of immediate injury, the presence of hematomas and edema, and the need for neurosurgical intervention.

9. MRI is a more sensitive modality for traumatic brain injury but often cannot be performed early in the patient's course because of neurologic, cardiovascular, or spinal instability. If done, it occasionally may pick up subacute or chronic subdural hematomas missed by CT scanning, as well as evidence of diffuse axonal injury (DAI), which is not usually visible on CT.

10. All patients with severe head injuries (Glasgow Coma Scale score of 8 or less) or major skull fractures require the early attention of a neurosurgeon. Deterioration in level of consciousness, intracranial hemorrhage, or focal neurologic findings demand immediate neurosurgical assessment.

11. If the patient is deteriorating, assume intracranial pressure is increased, administer mannitol and Lasix, and obtain a CT scan rapidly.

12. There is no role for steroids in the treatment of traumatic brain injury. A recent large randomized study showed no benefit upon mortality in over 10,000 patients randomized to steroids or placebo (level 1b evidence).

13. The value of *prophylactic antiepileptic drugs* after traumatic brain injury is unclear. Although phenytoin may decrease seizures in the first week after head injury, it may not decrease seizures over a longer period. With penetrating injuries or major hematoma, the risk of seizures is greater, suggesting that this group of patients is better suited for prophylactic therapy.

14. The *postconcussion syndrome* includes headache, dizziness, fatigue, decreased concentration, memory disorder, irritability, depression, and other psychological and somatic symptoms. In patients with such symptoms, medication (antidepressants) and rehabilitation may be helpful. Such patients may be difficult to treat if there are complicating social and litigation factors.

15. In some patients with persistent coma and a normal CT scan, diffuse axonal injury (DAI) is present. In these cases, shearing injury to axons is present. Coma of 6 to 24 hours duration is termed mild DAI, and coma of more than 24 hours is considered moderate to severe DAI, depending on the presence of brainstem signs. DAI is the most important cause of persistent disability after traumatic brain injury.

16. Many medications have been tried for behavioral modification after severe head injury. Patients with severe head injury may have agitation, irritability, depression, and occasionally aggressive behavior. There is limited evidence-based information to support any specific strategy or guideline for such care (grade C recommendation).

17. To date there is not sufficient evidence to support therapeutic hypothermia in head-injured patients.

Suggested Readings

Alderson P, Gadkary C, Signorini DF. Therapeutic hypothermia for head injury. *Cochrane Database*. 2004:CD001048.

CRASH trial collaborators. Effect of intravenous corticosteroids on death within 14 days in 10008 adults with clinically significant head injury (MRC CRASH trial): randomised placebo-controlled trial. *Lancet*. 2004;364:1321–1328.

Cushman JG, Agarwal N, Fabian TC, et al. Practice management guidelines for the management of mild traumatic brain injury: the EAST practice management guidelines work group. *J Trauma*. 2001;51:1016–1026.

Gupta AK. Monitoring the injured brain in the intensive care unit. *J Postgrad Med.* 2002;48:218–225.

Hammoud DA, Wasserman BA. Diffuse axonal injuries: pathophysiology and imaging. *Neuroimaging Clin North Am.* 2002;12:205–216.

Mazzola CA, Adelson PD. Critical care management of head trauma in children. *Crit Care Med.* 2002;30(suppl):S393–S401.

McDonald BC, Flashman LA, Saykin AJ. Executive dysfunction following traumatic brain injury: neural substrates and treatment strategies. *Neurorehabilitation.* 2002;17:333–344.

McNaughton H, Harwood M. Traumatic brain injury: assessment and management. *Hosp Med.* 2002;63:8–11.

National Collaborating Centre for Acute Care. *Head Injury: Triage, Assessment, Investigation and Early Management of Head Injury in Infants, Children and Adults.* London: National Institute for Clinical Excellence (NICE); 2003.

Neurobehavioral Guidelines Working Group. Guidelines for the pharmacologic treatment of neurobehavioral sequelae of traumatic brain injury. *J Neurotrauma.* 2006;23:1468–1501.

Zee CS, Hovanessian A, Go JL, et al. Imaging of sequelae of head trauma. *Neuroimaging Clin North Am.* 2002;12:325–338.

Neurodiagnostic Procedures

ELECTROENCEPHALOGRAM

The electroencephalogram (EEG) is a physiologic monitor of cortical function. It measures electrical activity that is generated in the cerebral cortex and then synchronized and modulated by thalamic and reticular activating structures. EEG is most useful in seizure disorders, encephalopathies, and coma.

1. *Seizure disorders*. The EEG is a key test for the diagnosis and management of patients with seizure disorders. It should be emphasized that not all patients with clinically definite seizure disorders have abnormalities on EEG, and conversely, paroxysmal EEG abnormalities sometimes are seen in people without seizure disorders. During a tonic-clonic seizure, an EEG usually demonstrates widespread electrical discharges. Interictally (i.e., between seizures, not during seizures), patients with complex partial seizures may have focal spikes, well-defined waves that are sharply contoured and localized in one or more areas. During a complex partial seizure, they may show a focal buildup of rhythmic waves. Simple partial seizures may not show abnormalities on the surface EEG at all. Interictal EEGs in patients with seizure disorders are abnormal in approximately 70% of patients. Certain seizure disorders are classified according to EEG patterns:
   - *Absence seizure*, a seizure characterized by brief losses of consciousness (e.g., staring spells of no more than several seconds), occurs almost exclusively in people between the ages of 5 and 18. It shows classic three-per-second spike-and-wave discharges. The diagnosis of absence seizures depends on this EEG finding.
   - *Temporal lobe epilepsy* is characterized by focal EEG abnormalities in either or both temporal lobes, including sharp waves or spike discharges. These abnormalities may not be apparent on routine interictal EEGs but usually can be demonstrated by sleep EEGs or by using special scalp leads over the temporal regions. If temporal lobe epilepsy is

suspected, such procedures should be carried out. Continuous monitoring may be necessary in difficult cases.

- *Lennox–Gastaut syndrome* is a childhood syndrome, often with mental retardation, in which patients have several seizure types. The interictal EEG shows characteristic slow spike-and-wave discharges. *West syndrome* is associated with early childhood seizures called infantile spasms and has a characteristic EEG pattern of high-voltage slow waves and spikes (hypsarrhythmia).
- The EEG is often useful in the decision of whether to discontinue anticonvulsant medication (see Chapter 20).

2. *Encephalopathy.* Patients with metabolic encephalopathy of any cause have abnormal EEGs, consisting of nonfocal slowing of the EEG pattern or rhythmic bursts of symmetric frontal slowing. The EEG can be useful in identifying metabolic encephalopathies or in ruling out metabolic encephalopathies in patients with altered mental status. Certain patterns can be helpful (e.g., the "triphasic" waves of hepatic encephalopathy).

3. *Coma.* For patients in a coma, the EEG can assist with identifying severe injury, subclinical seizure activity, or major asymmetries and may provide good prognostic signs such as the presence of reactivity and sleep potentials.

4. *Tumors.* Depending on the location and size of a tumor, the EEG is often abnormal, with focal slowing or spike discharges. New onset of seizures in middle age is often the presenting symptom of tumor. However, the CT scan or magnetic resonance imaging (MRI) is the major test used to diagnose tumors or other space-occupying lesions.

5. *Other diseases.* Some disorders have characteristic EEG findings (e.g., Creutzfeldt–Jakob disease, herpes simplex encephalitis, subacute sclerosing panencephalitis). Psychiatric diseases (affective disorders, schizophrenia) usually have no effect on the EEG. Migraine headaches may be associated with focal slowing. The EEG is often used as an adjunct in the diagnosis of brain death (isoelectric EEG).

ELECTROMYOGRAPHY

The electromyogram (EMG) is an electrical test measuring physiologic function in muscle. It is used to help diagnose muscle disease, disease of the neuromuscular junction, and denervation of muscles secondary to nerve, plexus, or root lesions. Specific abnormalities seen in EMG include alteration of the motor unit (increased size and duration in chronic denervation), fibrillation and positive sharp waves in acute denervation, and abnormal electrical excitability in metabolic disorders.

1. Patients with *myopathy* often show certain features: (i) low-amplitude, short-duration motor unit potentials; (ii) complex polyphasic motor unit potentials; and (iii) increased insertional activity (e.g., bizarre high-frequency discharges; usually seen with inflammatory myopathies). It is usually impossible to distinguish one myopathy from another by EMG. Some myopathies (e.g., polymyositis and muscular dystrophies) may show fibrillation potentials.

2. *Myotonia* presents a characteristic pattern of hyperexcitability with persistent waxing and waning and repetitive discharges, which sound like a "dive bomber." The dive bomber pattern is not diagnostic of any single myotonic disorder.

3. Presynaptic *neuromuscular junction (NMJ) disorders* (e.g., botulism, Eaton–Lambert syndrome) may be characterized by progressive enhancement of motor unit action potentials evoked by repetitive stimulation of the motor nerve. Most also show normal amplitude miniature end-plate potentials. By contrast, postsynaptic NMJ disorders (e.g., myasthenia gravis) show a decremental response of the muscle action potential with repetitive nerve stimulation and subnormal amplitudes of the miniature endplate potentials.

4. *Denervation* produces increased polyphasic action potentials, bizarre high-frequency discharges, fibrillations, positive sharp waves, and sometimes fasciculations. Fibrillation potentials develop 3 to 4 weeks after the onset of nerve injury. Thus, someone with an acute root or nerve lesion may not show muscle fibrillation. Examination of muscle groups in the legs or arms may help to diagnose specific root lesions and whether denervated muscles are referable to a single root. Similarly, denervation can be used to help diagnose amyotrophic lateral sclerosis or other anterior horn cell diseases.

NERVE CONDUCTION STUDIES

Nerve conduction studies yield information about the integrity of myelin and axon in peripheral nerve. If nerve conduction studies are abnormal in all limbs, a *generalized* neuropathy is implied (e.g., diabetic or alcoholic neuropathies). Disorders that primarily affect myelin (e.g., Guillain–Barré syndrome) cause nerve conduction slowing out of proportion to EMG changes, whereas "axonal" neu-ropathies (e.g., caused by alcohol) cause EMG changes of dener-vation in proportion to nerve conduction abnormalities. Individual nerve abnormalities can be seen in nerve entrapments (e.g., carpal tunnel) or nerve infarction or damage (e.g., mononeuritis multi-plex). Nerve conduction studies are useful in focal entrapment syndromes such as carpal tunnel syndrome and ulnar entrapment at the elbow.

EVOKED POTENTIALS

An evoked potential is an electrical response recorded from the CNS and elicited by an external stimulus, either visual, auditory, or somatosensory. Evoked potentials are useful in localizing sub-tle sensory lesions and in detecting unsuspected subclinical sen-sory deficits. With the advent of MRI scanning, the use of evoked potentials has diminished.

1. *Visual evoked responses* (VERs), measured over the occiput, are stimulated by the patient watching a shifting checkerboard pattern on a monitor. Normally they elicit a large amplitude response about 100 milliseconds after the stimulus. VERs are most helpful in demonstrating lesions in the optic nerves and are particularly useful in diagnosis of multiple sclerosis (MS).

2. *Brainstem auditory evoked responses* are elicited by delivering click stimuli to either ear. Their major advantage is the ability to localize auditory pathway lesions to eighth nerve, cochlear nucleus, superior olive, lateral lemniscus, or inferior colliculus. They are exquisitely sensitive to extrinsic lesions, such as acoustic neuromas, and may detect these lesions before they are visible by CT scan. They are also sensitive to intrinsic brain-stem lesions involving the auditory pathways as seen in MS, brainstem glioma, brainstem infarcts, and olivopontocerebellar degeneration. In MS, because there are other more sensitive methods of assessment, they are no longer being used as much as in the past. Because they are not abolished by high doses of anesthesia or barbiturates, they are useful monitors of brain-stem integrity in patients undergoing neurosurgical procedures on the posterior fossa.

3. *Somatosensory evoked responses* (SERs) are elicited by stimu-lating large-fiber sensory systems peripherally. Tibial and per-oneal evoked responses may help to localize lesions to their respective peripheral nerves, lumbosacral plexus, dorsal

spinal cord, spinomedullary junction, brainstem, and thalamus. Median nerve SERs will assess function along the arm and centrally through the cervical spine, brainstem, and thalamus. Pudendal SERs help to detect deficits of sensory innervation of the genitalia. Virtually any lesion compromising conduction in these systems (e.g., MS, spinal cord tumors, severe cervical spondylosis) may produce SER abnormalities. SERs are useful adjuncts to monitor spinal cord function during spinal surgery.

MAGNETIC RESONANCE IMAGING

Magnetic resonance imaging (MRI) is the imaging modality of choice for several neurologic disorders, including congenital anomalies, especially those involving the posterior fossa (e.g., Arnold–Chiari); pathology of the sella turcica, including pituitary tumors; lesions involving the internal auditory canal (e.g., acoustic neuroma); lesions of the posterior fossa, including brainstem and cerebellum (e.g., brainstem gliomas, cerebellar astrocytoma); lesions of temporal lobes and white matter diseases, especially those of demyelinating origin (e.g., MS); and spinal cord lesion (e.g., spinal cord tumors, syringomyelia). MRI has become an important part of the diagnosis of stroke and is used in refractory epilepsies to assess for cortical abnormalities.

An MRI scan takes approximately 30 to 60 minutes, and during most of this time, the patient must lie motionless. If this is impossible, sedation may be required. A scan consists of a pulsating magnetic field (heard as banging sounds by the patient) and a continuous high-strength magnetic field (which the patient does not feel). An MRI cannot be performed in patients with pacemakers, intracranial aneurysm clips, or a metallic foreign body in the eye or brain. Some intracranial clips and prosthetic heart valves may also be problematic.

Each patient needs to be carefully evaluated for his or her risk of MRI before undergoing the procedure.

Injected paramagnetic dye (gadolinium) may improve the yield when imaging for tumors or inflammatory disorders around the brain.

Patients with renal disease of significance may develop a potentially fatal dermopathy after the use of gadolinium (nephrogenic fibrosing dermopathy).

The areas of the nervous system where MRI has a particular advantage over CT are those where there is significant bony artifact (especially brainstem and spinal cord). MRI continues to have limitations when poor patient cooperation and movement precludes a prolonged period with the patient still in the study or when the issue is deciding whether acute hemorrhage has occurred (e.g., subarachnoid hemorrhage). Advances in software and in altering pulse sequences may resolve these problems in the future.

Points of particular interest with respect to MRI imaging of the nervous system include the following:

1. *Seizures.* MRI is the imaging modality of choice in the evaluation of patients with new-onset seizures. Its ability to image in three planes makes it more sensitive in detecting lesions that may cause seizures and in delineating their size and location. The coronal views are particularly valuable in detecting temporal lobe lesions. AVMs, neoplasms, or cortical dysplasias, as well as mesial temporal sclerosis, may be seen in epilepsy patients.

2. *Headaches.* MRI is valuable in the evaluation of patients with new-onset or progressive headaches because of its ability to detect brain tumor, AVM, cerebral venous thrombosis, subdural hematomas, aneurysms, or hydrocephalus.

3. *Stroke.* CT remains the imaging modality of choice in the setting of acute stroke to exclude the presence of hemorrhage. MRI is more sensitive than CT (i) in the subacute stage to detect subtle hemorrhage; (ii) in imaging small infarctions, especially within the first 48 hours after symptom onset; (iii) in detecting infarctions in the posterior fossa; (iv) in detecting other lesions masquerading as stroke, such as brain tumor; and (v) in detecting cavernous sinus thrombosis.

4. *Head trauma.* CT remains the appropriate study in the acute evaluation of the trauma patient in searching for an extra-axial blood clot or assessing acute brain damage and acute skull injury using bone windows. MRI is preferred in the subacute state to detect extra-axial hematoma, contusion, and shearing injury.

5. *Dementia.* MRI is valuable in evaluation of the patient with dementia because of its ability to detect and delineate tumors, subdural hematoma, multiple infarcts, and cerebral atrophy.

6. *Multiple sclerosis.* MRI is useful in demonstrating the demyelinating lesions of MS. Patients without clinical evidence of brain involvement (e.g., when presenting with optic neuritis or a spinal cord lesion) frequently are found to have characteristic periventricular lesions on MRI. Gadolinium enhancement shows plaques are active and may influence treatment decisions.

7. *Spine and spinal cord.* MRI is the imaging examination of choice for disorders that affect the spine or spinal cord. It is of particular value for visualizing primary spinal cord tumors (e.g., gliomas), intradural or extradural processes dial impinge

on the spinal cord (e.g., meningiomas, metastatic tumors), syringomyelia, hematomyelia, and spinal stenosis.

8. *Congenital anomalies.* MRI is an excellent modality to demonstrate congenital anomalies, such as Dandy–Walker cyst in the posterior fossa, Arnold–Chiari malformation, and agenesis of the corpus callosum. It provides details of abnormal morphology in the dysmorphic brain (e.g., in derangements of myelination).

MAGNETIC RESONANCE ANGIOGRAPHY

Magnetic resonance angiography (MRA) is a technique that noninvasively images the blood vessels. The flow void seen in blood vessels is reconstructed, allowing an evaluation of the intracranial and extracranial vessels. MRA is limited in that the image may be degraded by movement and by tortuous flow in vessels, which will show up as a gap in magnetic resonance signal. However, MRA helps assess vessel stenosis, large aneurysms, AVMs, and venous sinus disease.

COMPUTED TOMOGRAPHY SCAN

Computerized axial tomography heralded a revolution in the diagnosis and management of neurologic disease. Its use lessened with the development of MRI but has reemerged with the advent of CT angiography.

Contrast enhancement in CT scanning generally is used to assist diagnosis of certain infections and tumors. The danger of "routine" contrast use relates to allergy to the dye and the effect of dye on renal function. The decision to use contrast rests on the clinical circumstances. Contrast should be avoided in patients with marginal renal function and should be used with caution in dehydrated patients with diabetes because of the risk of renal failure.

1. *Cerebrovascular disease.* The basic value of the CT scan in cerebrovascular disease is to differentiate hemorrhage from infarction. Virtually all hemorrhages show up as increased density on CT scans, whereas either no abnormality or decreased density is seen with infarction. This distinction is particularly important because it is impossible to distinguish infarction from hemorrhage on clinical grounds alone. No patient should be anticoagulated without prior CT scan to rule out bleeding. Of infarcts, 15% to 20% are apparent immediately on CT scan, and most moderate-sized infarcts are apparent at 3 to 5 days.

The diagnosis of multiple infarcts caused by emboli also can be made by CT scan, including infarcts seen in areas that have not declared themselves clinically. CT scan can identify AVMs and aneurysms, although the precise diagnosis of these disorders usually requires arteriography.

2. *Tumors.* Virtually all tumors larger than 2 to 4 mm can be seen on CT scan. Depending on the pattern, certain diagnostic interpretations can be made. CT scan sensitivity to tumors is enhanced by perfusion with iodinated contrast agents.

3. *Hydrocephalus.* Although CT scan and MRI are useful for the demonstration of hydrocephalus, MRI is more accurate in determining the cause (e.g., aqueductal stenosis).

4. *Degenerative disease.* Patients with CNS degenerative diseases, such as Alzheimer disease, usually have normal CT scan early in the disease. However, as patients get older, they usually have widened sulci and enlarged ventricles because of loss of brain tissue. Brain atrophy does not necessarily correlate with dementia and also can be seen in "normal" people. There are patients with degenerative disease or dementia who have normal-appearing CT scans.

5. *Subdural hematoma.* Approximately 80% of subdural hematomas, both unilateral and bilateral, can be seen on CT scan. Some subdurals may be isodense and not visualized by CT scan. These may be seen with contrast injection or with MRI scanning.

6. *Trauma.* CT is effective in differentiating many consequences of trauma in the nervous system, including fractures, epidural and subdural hematomas, and shifts of intracranial contents. CT scanning is an excellent screening method for showing intracranial shifts before performing LP.

7. CT angiography is a technique using computerized timing of injected dye to image the aortic arch, the carotids, and the intracranial structures. It may be used as a rapid method to analyze the vascular system and is being used to assess patients with acute cerebral infarction. Its use is limited by the computer analysis required for interpretation, the high dye load of iodinated dye, and the relatively large radiation dose, which may be a concern with multiple repeated scans.

ARTERIOGRAPHY

Cerebral arteriography is used to define vascular disease of intracranial and extracranial vessels (e.g., carotid artery disease, AVM, and aneurysms) when less invasive procedures are inconclusive. MRA obviates the need for arteriography in many cases. For some diseases, such as the evaluation of small berry aneurysms and cerebral vasculitis, angiography remains more sensitive than MRA. Risks of arteriography include reaction to the contrast media, thrombosis or hemorrhage at the catheter introduction site, arrhythmia, transient global amnesia, seizure, and stroke. The risks of arteriography must be weighed against the benefits, particularly with the variety of alternative noninvasive procedures that are available.

CAROTID ULTRASOUND AND TRANSCRANIAL DOPPLER

Carotid ultrasound is a noninvasive technique that, in expert operator hands, has a high sensitivity and specificity for carotid disease. It is used most commonly to screen for the presence of moderate or severe carotid stenosis due to atherosclerosis. In addition it may be helpful in carotid dissection due to trauma or spontaneous dissection. Transcranial Doppler is a technique of focusing a Doppler signal at different depths through windows at the base of the skull or through the skull itself. It may show evidence for intracranial stenosis or reversal of flow due to vascular disease. It has also been used in the confirmation of cerebral death. It has most recently been used to diagnosis and follow up vasospasm related to subarachnoid hemorrhage, and can be done repeatedly in the ICU setting. It has also been used therapeutically as an adjunct to thrombolytic therapy for acute stroke.

Suggested Readings

Caruso G, Eisen A, Stalberg E, et al. Clinical EMG and glossary of terms most commonly used by clinical electromyographers. The international federation of clinical neurophysiology. *EEG Clin Neurophysiol.* 1999;52(suppl):189–198.

Flink R, Pedersen B, Guekht AB, et al. Guidelines for the use of EEG methodology in the diagnosis of epilepsy. *Acta Neurol Scand.* 2002;106:1–7.

Gronseth GS, Ashman EJ. Practice parameter: the usefulness of evoked potentials in identifying clinically silent lesions in patients with suspected multiple sclerosis (an evidence-based review): report of the Quality Standards Subcommittee of the American Academy of Neurology. *Neurology.* 2000;54: 1720–1725.

Practice parameter for electrodiagnostic studies in carpal tunnel syndrome: summary statement. *Muscle Nerve*. 2002;25:918–922.

Wardlaw JM, Chappell FM, Best JJ, et al. Non-invasive imaging compared with intra-arterial angiography in the diagnosis of symptomatic carotid stenosis: a meta-analysis. *Lancet*. 2006; 367:1503–1512.

34 Key Points in Neuroanatomy

The examination of the nervous system depends on knowledge of the anatomy, which underlies the clinical findings. Following are some key points of neuroanatomy to help localize and diagnose neurologic disorders.

CEREBRAL CORTEX

The cerebral cortex comprises of four lobes for each hemisphere and each lobe has specialized functions (Fig. 34.1).

1. *Frontal* lobes participate in speech (the Broca area for speech is in the dominant hemisphere), movement (corticospinal tracts originate here), personality, and initiative. Frontal eye fields participate in conjugate eye deviation, so that lesions on one side cause the eye to deviate to the ipsilateral side. Signs of frontal disease: Broca aphasia (dominant), altered personality, utilization behavior (picks up and uses objects aimlessly), perseveration, altered judgment, apathy (abulia), apraxia, motor impersistence (give up on tasks, usually nondominant).

2. *Temporal* lobes participate in memory functions and auditory processing. For language, it is the dominant hemisphere; for music, it is usually the nondominant hemisphere. A unilateral temporal lesion may cause a contralateral superior quadrantanopsia as a result of involvement of optic radiations. Temporal lobe lesions may also cause memory loss; Kluver–Bucy syndrome (bilateral temporal lesions) of hyperorality, disinhibition of sexuality, hyperphagia; pure word deafness (can hear noises, but cannot understand speech, can read and speak normally), or Wernicke aphasia (dominant).

3. *Parietal* cortex participates in sensation, thus contralateral loss of cortical sensation occurs with lesions (two-point discrimination, identification of objects or numbers drawn in the hand). A mild hemiparesis may occur with parietal injury. Alexia, agraphia, left/right discrimination difficulty, and finger naming difficulty occur with a lesion in the left angular gyrus

CEREBRAL CORTEX

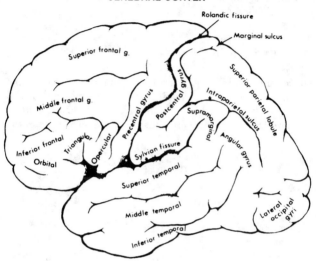

FIGURE 34.1. Left hemisphere showing frontal, parietal, temporal, and occipital lobes. (Reproduced with permission of Ms. Linda Wilson-Pauwels and B.C. Decker, Inc., Hamilton, Ontario, Canada.)

of the parietal lobe (dominant hemisphere). Nondominant parietal lesions may cause visuospatial difficulty, dressing apraxia, a loss of awareness of the left side of the body, and topographic memory loss. Parietal lesions may also cause constructional apraxia (difficulty copying figures), ideomotor apraxia (inability to show motor acts such as throwing a ball, brushing their teeth), neglect (either of one side of body or one side of space). Nondominant parietal lesions may also cause an unawareness of a deficit on the opposite side of the body (anosognosia) and blunting of emotional responses or awareness of emotionality in others (aprosody).

4. *Occipital* lobes participate in vision. Lesions of the occipital lobe cause visual field loss, hallucinosis, or blindness. Altered recognition of objects or faces by sight also may occur. Patients with bilateral occipital lobe infarctions may be cortically blind (papillary reflexes are intact) but unaware of their blindness (Anton syndrome). Occipital lesions may also cause homonymous scotomas, visual hallucinations, palinopsia (image repeated more than once), prosopagnosia: difficulty naming faces, distortions of visual images, loss of color vision, or alexia

without agraphia (dominant lesion occipital lobe and posterior corpus callosum).

CIRCLE OF WILLIS

The anterior, middle, and posterior cerebral arteries supply the anteromesial cortex; the lateral frontal, temporal, and parietal lobes; and the occipital lobes, respectively. The internal carotid, and anterior and middle cerebral arteries are referred to as the

Circle of Willis

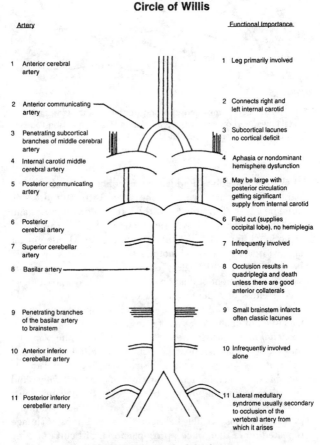

Artery	Functional Importance
1 Anterior cerebral artery	1 Leg primarily involved
2 Anterior communicating artery	2 Connects right and left internal carotid
3 Penetrating subcortical branches of middle cerebral artery	3 Subcortical lacunes no cortical deficit
4 Internal carotid middle cerebral artery	4 Aphasia or nondominant hemisphere dysfunction
5 Posterior communicating artery	5 May be large with posterior circulation getting significant supply from internal carotid
6 Posterior cerebral artery	6 Field cut (supplies occipital lobe). no hemiplegia
7 Superior cerebellar artery	7 Infrequently involved alone
8 Basilar artery	8 Occlusion results in quadriplegia and death unless there are good anterior collaterals
9 Penetrating branches of the basilar artery to brainstem	9 Small brainstem infarcts often classic lacunes
10 Anterior inferior cerebellar artery	10 Infrequently involved alone
11 Posterior inferior cerebellar artery	11 Lateral medullary syndrome usually secondary to occlusion of the vertebral artery from which it arises

FIGURE 34.2. Cerebral circulation.

anterior circulation. The basilar artery supplies the upper brain-stem, and the vertebral arteries supply the lower brainstem and cerebellum. These together are referred to as the posterior circulation. The anastomotic circle of Willis connects the anterior and posterior circulation through the posterior communicating arteries and the left and right circulations through the anterior communicating artery. The circle of Willis is frequently anatomically incomplete (Fig. 34.2).

EYE MOVEMENTS IN NEUROLOGIC DISEASE

The frontal eye fields exert a major influence on horizontal eye movement, each field being concerned with contralateral eye deviation. Thus, the right field causes eyes to move to the left. (The fibers cross in the pons and connect there to the extraocular muscles via the medial longitudinal fasciculus.) Both fields are constantly active, striking a balance; thus, when one is more or less active than the other, horizontal eye deviation results (Fig. 34.3).

A *destructive lesion* in the hemisphere or subcortex causes eyes to deviate toward the same side as the lesion. Thus, with a right-sided lesion, the eyes are deviated to the right. An excitatory lesion at the cortical level (e.g., a seizure) causes eyes to deviate to the contralateral side. A *destructive lesion* in the pons causes eyes to deviate to the side opposite the damage. Thus, with a left-sided lesion, eyes deviate to the right. Eye deviation secondary to hemisphere lesions, but not brainstem lesions, may be overcome by brainstem reflexes (e.g., doll's eye maneuver).

Horizontal eye movements are served by the medial (third nerve) and lateral (sixth nerve) rectus muscles (Fig. 34.4). Inputs from the cortex and eighth nerve nuclei affect the paramedian pontine reticular formation, which drives the sixth nerve nucleus. This stimulates the ipsilateral lateral rectus and contralateral medial rectus, connecting with the latter through the medial longitudinal fasciculus. A lesion in the sixth nerve nucleus causes a paralysis of ipsilateral gaze (cannot bring the eyes to the side injured because of weakness in the ipsilateral lateral rectus and contralateral medial rectus).

Vertical eye movements are organized in the midbrain in a variety of nuclei. Thus disorders of up- and down-gaze suggest a midbrain lesion, and altered horizontal gaze suggests a pontine lesion. Convergence is also located in the midbrain and patients with midbrain lesions may have a combination of altered vertical gaze and loss of convergence.

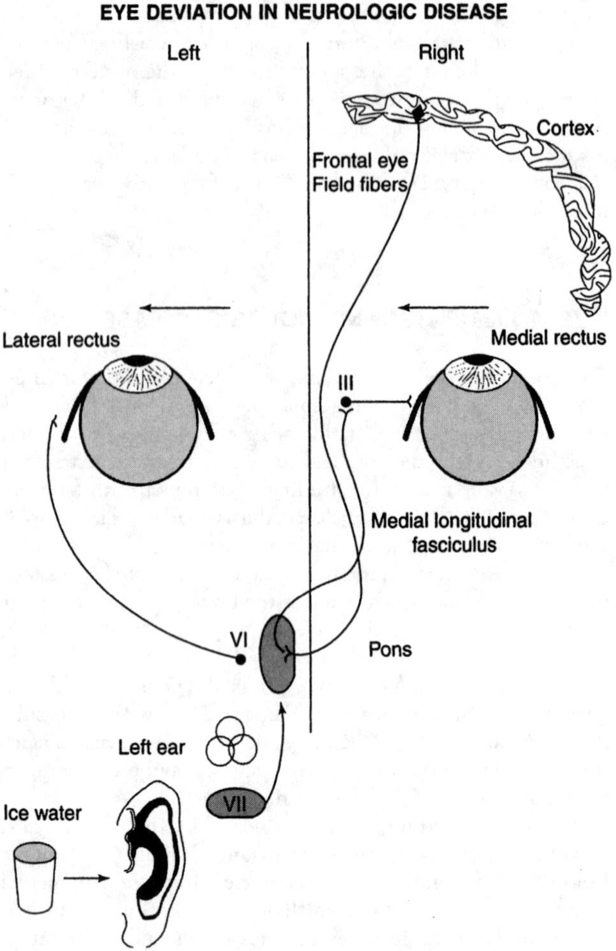

EYE DEVIATION IN NEUROLOGIC DISEASE

FIGURE 34.3. In the comatose patient with an intact brainstem, ice water in the left ear causes deviation of the eyes to the left.

Various Eye Signs and What They May Indicate

There are a number of eye signs in neurology and each of them may suggest certain localizations or pathologies. For this reason it's worth knowing the specific syndromes and what they may suggest.

- *Periodic alternating nystagmus:* In the primary position (straight ahead) eyes beat to one side for a few seconds to a minute, slow

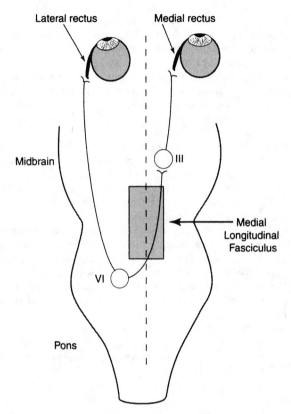

FIGURE 34.4. Horizontal eye movements.

and stop beating, then begin to beat to the opposite side. This alternates every 2 minutes with a regular cycle. Indicates lesion of the flocculonodular lobe of the cerebellum, which may respond to lioresal.

- *Upbeating nystagmus:* Jerk nystagmus evoked by upgaze. Seen in a variety of brainstem and cerebellar lesions, so localizes to the posterior fossa.
- *Downbeat nystagmus:* Jerk nystagmus evoked by down gaze or seen in the primary position. Suggests lesion of the cervicomedullary junction, commonly seen in Arnold–Chiari malformations.
- *Pendular nystagmus:* A non-jerk nystagmus with a side-to-side or up-and-down motion with equal excursions back and forth.

Seen in a variety of conditions, typical of congenital nystagmus (horizontal pendular nystagmus). Congenital nystagmus is a horizontal pendular nystagmus that has a null point just off of primary position to one side where nystagmus disappears.

- *Elliptical nystagmus:* A combination of pendular nystagmus in both horizontal and vertical directions that are out of phase causing a rotatory movement that can be circular or elliptical. A variety of brainstem conditions cause this, and it may be seen commonly in multiple sclerosis.
- *Internuclear opthalmoparesis:* In the primary position the eyes are OK, but when looking away from side affected the adducting eye either does not adduct or lags behind the abducting eye, and the abducting eye has a gaze-evoked jerk nystagmus. May be bilateral. Lesions of medial longitudinal fasciculus in pons or midbrain, midline pontine lesions.
- *Opsoclonus:* Sudden large amplitude conjugate eye movements in various directions. May be due to cerebellar disease. May be seen in some paraneoplastic conditions, occasionally associated with myoclonus (opsoclonus-myoclonus syndrome).
- *Ocular flutter:* In primary position eyes suddenly have a rapid, jiggling motion in the horizontal plane lasting a second, occurring intermittently. Brainstem lesions.
- *Rebound nystagmus:* On gazing in one direction eyes have a gaze-evoked nystagmus to that side that gradually reduces. On return to primary position eyes rebound to beat in the opposite direction. Cerebellar lesions.

VISUAL PATHWAYS (FIG. 34.5)

1. *Blindness in one eye* represents retinal or ipsilateral optic nerve dysfunction. The optic nerve is frequently involved in multiple sclerosis (optic neuritis), producing unilateral blindness or a central loss of vision (scotoma); it also may be involved by tumor (optic glioma) or undergo atrophy secondary to prolonged increased intracranial pressure. The optic nerve also may be affected by vascular processes such as giant-cell arteritis and amaurosis fugax.
2. *Bitemporal hemianopsia* is found classically in pituitary tumor secondary to pressure on the optic chiasm. Non-homonymous field defects usually imply lesions near the chiasm. Remember, concentric tunnel vision may be seen in hysterical blindness.
3. *Homonymous hemianopsia* implies a lesion posterior to the chiasm. It may involve optic tract or optic radiations emanating

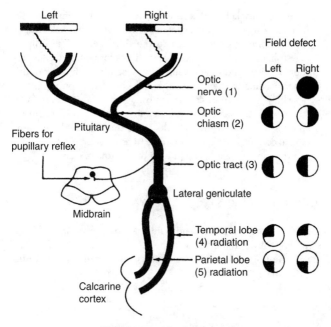

FIGURE 34.5. Visual pathways.

from the lateral geniculate body (or the lateral geniculate itself). The closer a lesion is to the lateral geniculate, the smaller it can be and still produce a homonymous hemianopsia. Occlusions of the posterior cerebral artery usually produce homonymous hemianopsia with sparing of the macula.

4. The *optic radiations* fan out from the lateral geniculate and travel in the temporal and parietal lobes before reaching their destination in the occipital lobe. Lesions in the temporal lobe may give a homonymous superior field defect if the optic radiations are affected. Similarly, a lesion in the parietal lobe may show a homonymous inferior field defect.

5. When one realizes the large territory needed for intact visual fields, it becomes apparent why checking visual fields is a mandatory part of every neurologic examination.

6. With *pupillary response* the pupil depends on input from both the parasympathetic nervous system via the third cranial nerves and sympathetic inputs. Lesions of the third nerve cause dilation of the third nerve; lesion of the sympathetics cause constriction.

The pupillary light reflex has an afferent supply from the optic nerve, through the lateral geniculate nucleus of the thalamus, to the midbrain pretectal area to the third nerve. The Ediger-Westphal nucleus supplies efferent fibers for papillary constriction. Horner syndrome is caused by sympathetic disorder of the fibers leading to the pupil and face. Miosis (small pupil), ptosis (partial), and anhidrosis (caused by sweat gland innervation to the face on the same side) are seen in combination. The sympathetics travel from the hypothalamus through the brainstem, spinal cord to T1 or 2, out the roots to near the apex of the lung, up the carotid sheath, and in with the ophthalmic artery.

CRANIAL NERVES

Remember, the first and second cranial nerves lie outside the brainstem. The third and fourth are in the midbrain, fifth through eighth are in the pons, and ninth through twelfth are in the medulla (Fig. 34.6).

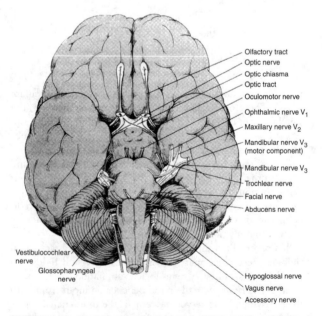

FIGURE 34.6. Cranial nerves. (Reproduced with permission of Ms. Linda Wilson-Pauwels and B.C. Decker, Inc., Hamilton, Ontario, Canada.)

I—olfactory, in medial cortex; rhinencephalon. Smell.

II—optic nerve, enters at lateral geniculate body. Visual function.

III—oculomotor nerve; midbrain. Innervates medial, superior, and inferior rectus; inferior oblique; lid elevator; and pupil.

IV—trochlear nerve; midbrain. Innervates superior oblique, brings eye down and in.

V—trigeminal; pons (and medulla). Supplies muscles of mastication, facial sensation, corneal reflex.

VI—abducens; pons. Supplies lateral rectus, brings eye outward.

VII—facial. Supplies facial movements, tearing, and salivation.

VIII—auditory. Supplies hearing and vestibular function.

IX—glossopharyngeal. Supplies palatal sensation.

X—vagus. Supplies muscles of swallowing, autonomic parasympathetics to internal organs.

XI—spinal accessory nerve. Supplies sternocleidomastoid and trapezius muscles.

XII—hypoglossal. Supplies muscles of the tongue.

MIDBRAIN

The most prominent disturbance in the midbrain (cranial nerves III to IV) generally involves the third nerve nucleus or exiting fibers, producing a dilated pupil and ophthalmoplegia (Fig. 34.7). Lesions affecting the area of the midbrain just below the superior colliculus produce difficulty with upward gaze, convergence, and pupillary light reflexes (Parinaud syndrome). A tumor pressing on the superior colliculus may present in this way (e.g., pinealoma).

Midbrain (Cranial Nerves III to IV).

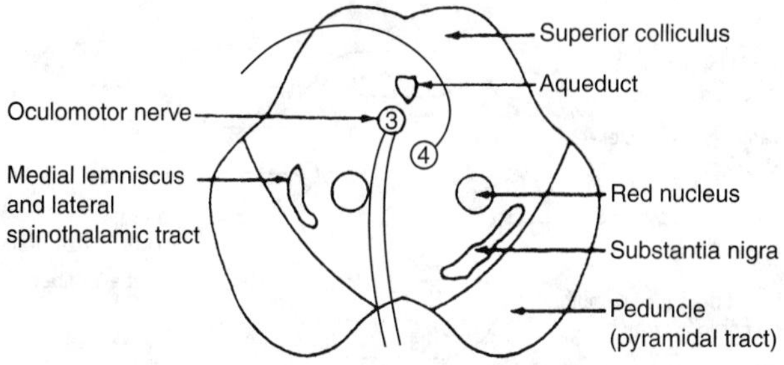

FIGURE 34.7. Midbrain.

Lesions of the red nucleus produce contralateral ataxia and tremor (rubral tremor). The substantia nigra is located at this level and plays an important role in Parkinson disease.

The fourth nerve nucleus also is located in the midbrain at a lower level and seldom is involved alone. When it is involved alone (e.g., because of trauma), fourth nerve injury causes a head tilt.

Fibers from the optic tract are concerned with the pupillary response synapse in the region of the third nerve nucleus. Lesions in the midbrain may impair pupillary reaction to direct light but leave contraction to accommodation intact.

PONS

The fibers of the seventh (facial) nerve sweep around the sixth nerve (lateral rectus) before exiting from the pons (cranial nerves V to VIII) (Fig. 34.8). Thus, a lesion at this level often produces a VI and VII nerve paralysis on the same side.

In the basic structure of the pons, medial involvement produces motor dysfunction and internuclear ophthalmoplegia or gaze palsy to the side of the lesion. Lateral involvement causes pain and temperature dysfunction.

Vertical nystagmus is a sign of brainstem dysfunction at the level of the pontomedullary junction or upper midbrain (unless the patient is taking barbiturates). Eighth nerve nuclei include cochlear and vestibular components.

The *trigeminal nerve* exits from the middle of the pons and if involved at this level produces face pain and ipsilateral loss of the corneal reflex. In high pontine lesions, pain and sensory loss are contralateral to the lesion in the face and extremities. Below the high pons, pain and temperature senses are lost ipsilaterally in the face and contralaterally in the limbs.

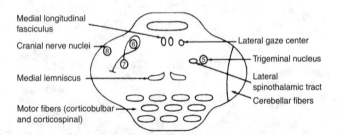

FIGURE 34.8. Pons (Cranial Nerves V to VIII).

Lesions of the *medical longitudinal fasciculus* (MLF) result in an internuclear ophthalmoplegia. If the right MLF is involved, there is difficulty with right eye adduction, as well as nystagmus in the abducting left eye when the patient looks to the left.

MEDULLA

The most commonly encountered vascular syndrome affecting the medulla (cranial nerves IX to XII) is the *lateral medullary* (*Wallenberg syndrome*) (see Chapter 16), which defines a major portion of the dysfunction that can be seen with medullary involvement (Fig. 34.9). (Medial structures are unaffected: pyramids, medial lemniscus, and twelfth nerve nucleus.) Cranial nerve nuclei include the following:

- *Twelfth (hypoglossal):* Unilateral involvement of nucleus causes fasciculations on that side; when the tongue is protruded, it deviates to the side of the lesion.
- *Tenth (vagus) and ninth (glossopharyngeal):* These innervate the laryngeal and pharyngeal musculature; dysphagia is prominent when they are involved.

Wallenberg Syndrome

Wallenberg syndrome: Lateral medulla.
Spinal tract of V: ipsilateral facial pinprick and temperature loss.
Vestibular nucleus: Vertigo, nystagmus, vomiting.
IX, X: ipsilateral palatal paralysis, dysarthria.

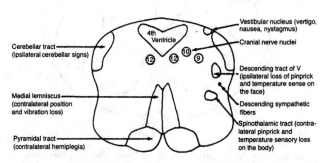

FIGURE 34.9. Medulla (Cranial Nerves IX to XII).

Sympathetics: ipsilateral Horner syndrome.
Restiform body: ipsilateral ataxia.

Remember that the *seventh (facial) nerve is not in the medulla*. Thus, if facial weakness is present, there must be dysfunction at the level of the pons or above.

SPINAL CORD

Vascular Supply

The *anterior spinal artery* (5) supplies the entire cord except for the dorsal columns. Thus, the anterior spinal artery syndrome produces paralysis and loss of pain and temperature sense; position and vibratory sense are preserved (Fig. 34.10).

The clinical correlation follows:

- Subacute combined system disease affects 1 and 3.
- Amyotrophic lateral sclerosis affects 3 and 4.
- Tabes dorsalis affects 1.
- Multiple sclerosis affects 1, 2, and 3 (alone or in combination).
- Poliomyelitis affects 4.
- Brown–Séquard syndrome (hemisection of cord) produces ipsilateral paralysis, ipsilateral loss of vibration and position sense, and contralateral loss of sensation to pinprick and temperature.

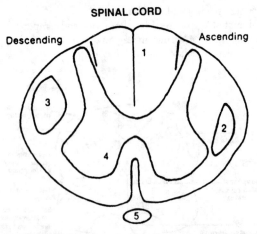

FIGURE 34.10. Spinal cord cross-section: 1. Dorsal columns. 2. Spinothalamic tracts; 3. Corticospinal tracts; 4. Anterior horns; 5. Anterior spinal artery.

Dorsal columns (1) carry position and vibratory sense; fibers rise ipsilaterally and cross in the medulla. These columns are laminated, but the lamination is usually of little clinical importance.

Lateral spinothalamic tract (2) carries pain and temperature sensation. These fibers cross on entering the cord; a cord lesion affecting them produces a contralateral loss. They are laminated with sacral fibers most laterally placed. Thus, an expanding process in the center of the cord gives sacral sparing (pinprick and temperature sensory loss are least prominent in the sacral area).

Descending Tracts

Lateral corticospinal tract (3) carries motor fibers that synapse at the anterior horn cells. The fibers have crossed in the medulla already. A lesion or pressure on the corticospinal tract causes weakness, spasticity, hyperreflexia, and upgoing toes.

Anterior horn cells (4) are lower motor neurons. A lesion here produces weakness, muscle wasting, fasciculations, and loss of reflexes and tone (Fig. 34.11).

See Table 34.1 for important crossings in the nervous system.

Suggested Readings

Adams RD, Victor M, Ropper AH. *Principles of Neurology*. 6th ed. New York: McGraw-Hill; 1997.

Brazis PW, Masdeu JC, Biller J. *Localization in Clinical Neurology*. 5th ed. Philadelphia: Williams & Wilkins; 2007.

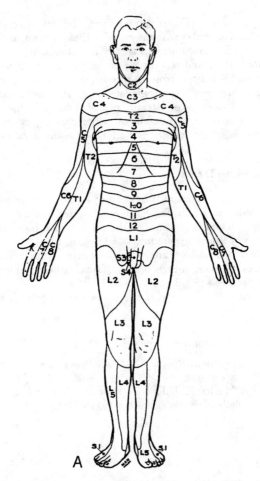

FIGURE 34.11. Dermatome sensory chart. **A.** Anterior view. (From Keegan JJ, Garrett FD. The segmental distribution of the cutaneous nerves in the limbs of man. *Anat Rec.* 1948;102:409. Reprinted with permission of Wiley-Liss, Inc., a subsidiary of John Wiley & Sons, Inc.)

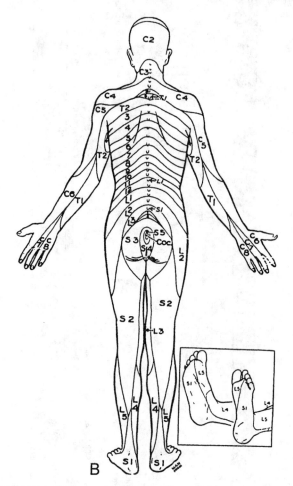

FIGURE 34.11. *(Continued)* **B.** Posterior view. (From Keegan JJ, Garrett FD. The segmental distribution of the cutaneous nerves in the limbs of man. *Anat Rec.* 1948;102:409. Reprinted with permission of Wiley-Liss, Inc., a subsidiary of John Wiley & Sons, Inc.)

■ **TABLE 34.1. Crossings in the Nervous System**[a]

Pathway	Function	Crosses	Interpretation
Pyramidal tract	Motor	Lower medulla	Lesion below crossing gives ipsilateral signs
Spinothalamic tract	Pain and temperature (body)	On entry to spinal cord	Lesion is always contralateral to pain and temperature loss (except in face)
Spinal tract of fifth (V) nerve	Pain and temperature (face)	Midpons (runs throughout medulla)	If lesion is in medulla or lower pons—ipsilateral loss; above midpons—contralateral loss
Spinal dorsal columns	Position and vibration	Lower medulla	Lesion below crossing gives ipsilateral signs
Cerebellar tracts	Coordination of movement	Crosses twice (on entry to cerebellum and in midbrain)	Because of the "double crossing" lesion of cerebellum or cerebellar tracts, usually produce signs and symptoms ipsilateral to lesion
Gaze fibers	Coordinates lateral gaze	Midpons	See Figure 34.2 for interpretation
Cranial nerve fibers	Cranial nerves	Just above cranial nerve	Lesion is ipsilateral when cranial nerve nuclei are involved

[a]Almost all major pathways in the nervous system cross. Much of the understanding of neuroanatomy relates to knowing where these tracts cross and, thus, at which level the nervous system is involved.

Differential Diagnoses in Neurology

Although long lists of differential diagnoses are usually unhelpful in clinical neurology, certain signs and symptoms suggest a list of diagnoses. This chapter includes selected topics that are not specifically mentioned in the text but have been found to be useful.

- **Amnesia, acute:** Head injury, postictal amnesia, transient global amnesia, encephalitis, intoxications (e.g., alcohol), basilar migraine, Wernicke encephalopathy, psychiatric.
- **Brachial plexus lesions:** Idiopathic brachial plexitis, tumor infiltration, trauma, radiation plexopathy, postinjection, polyarteritis nodosa, lupus, Lyme disease.
- **Choreoathetosis:** Huntington disease, Sydenham chorea, birth control pills, pregnancy associated (chorea gravidarum), stroke—basal ganglia, lupus, cerebral palsy, carbon monoxide, Sinemet, other dopamine agonists, Wilson disease.
- **Cranial nerve palsies:** Cavernous sinus lesion, base-of-skull disorders, meningeal disorders, idiopathic cranial neuropathy, intrinsic brainstem lesions, vasculitis, carotid dissection, myasthenia gravis.
- **Fasciculations:** Motor neuron disease, chronic root compression, benign fasciculation syndrome, polio, syringomyelia, metabolic disorders (thyrotoxicosis).
- **Horner syndrome:** Brainstem lesion, lower trunk brachial plexus lesion (apex of lung), cord lesion, neck lesion, carotid lesion, hypothalamic lesion.
- **Myelopathy:**
  Acute: Epidural metastases, ischemic, embolic, trauma, lupus, vasculitis, toxins (arsenic), multiple sclerosis (MS), arteriovenous malformation—with bleed, transverse myelitis.
  Chronic: MS, slow-growing tumors, primary lateral sclerosis, deficiencies (e.g., vitamin B_{12}), spinal stenosis.
- **Myoclonus:** Some epilepsies, anoxia, uremia, meningitis, encephalitis, cephalosporins and penicillins in patients with renal failure, gabapentin in renal failure patients or in high doses.
- **Recurrent meningitis:** Mollaret meningitis, bacterial with compromised barriers (cerebrospinal fluid leak, dural sinus),

parameningeal focus, drug induced (nonsteroidal medication), chemical, chemotherapy.

- **Neuropathy with "burning feet":** Diabetes, toxins including drugs, human immunodeficiency virus associated.
- **Ptosis:** Sympathetic lesion, migraine, cluster headache, myopathy, congenital ptosis, third-nerve lesion, redundant eyelid folds.
- **"Wasted hands":** Motor neuron disorders, plexus lesions (lower trunk), cervical root lesion, compression neuropathies (e.g., carpal tunnel), syringomyelia, distal myopathies.
- **White spots on the MRI:** MS, vascular disease, associated with migraine, MELAS, leukodystrophies, CNS lymphoma, CNS Sjögren syndrome, sarcoidosis, vitamin B_{12} deficiency.

Evidence-Based Medicine in Neurology

Over the past 20 years more attention has been given to the quality of evidence underlying medical decision making. While each discipline in medicine may have different disease entities and treatments for these diseases, basic approaches to analyzing diagnostic tests, prognosis, medications, and surgical interventions cross disciplinary lines. The science of designing, implementing, and evaluating the outcomes of clinical research falls under the rubric of evidence-based medicine, a term coined by physicians at McMaster University in Canada to emphasize the primacy of excellent-quality evidence in determining medical decisions.

In the past much of medical teaching revolved around teaching the experience of senior physicians during an apprenticeship period. It has become clear that the observation of individual patients and outcomes, while important in medical care, can be deceiving in terms of understanding the efficacy of medical interventions such as surgical therapies, medications, clinical practices, and so forth. Clinical trials design has become more sophisticated in an attempt to provide data that are as free of various biases as possible, and that when reviewed by experts in an area and experts in trial design can be judged to be valid and a true measure of efficacy for that population.

It also has been shown that theoretical approaches to disease management, such as extrapolating from animal model results, or using pathophysiologic approaches, are rife with error. Patients are not lab animals and randomized trials may not reproduce how we cogitate about disease entities. Time and time again randomized trials have produced results that would have been counter-intuitive but that are scientifically robust in nature.

Although it is beyond the scope of this text to fully review evidence-based medicine, it may be useful to have a description of approaches to analyzing the medical literature.

For diagnostic tests:

1. Has this test been analyzed in a patient sample that is representative of the spectrum of disease and types of patients that would be analyzed in a real world setting?
2. Is there a "gold standard" that this test is compared to independently and in a blind fashion?

3. If used, does this test change practice in some positive fashion (e.g., speed diagnosis, reduce costs, reduce inconvenience, reduce pain, improve sensitivity or specificity of diagnosis, lead to improvement of treatments, etc.)?

For treatment studies:

1. Were patients randomly assigned to treatment or comparison groups? Was there allocation bias? Were the patients representative of the ultimate target treatment group?
2. Were all patients entered in the study accounted for at the end of the study?
3. Were the outcomes significantly different between treatment and comparison groups? Were these differences clinically important?
4. Is the cost, inconvenience, side effect profile, or other operational features of the treatment worth it for the outcome change?
5. Were the outcomes measured in patient-oriented parameters that mattered (death, morbidity, patient satisfaction, cost, etc.) rather than disease-oriented outcomes (blood pressure, blood urea nitrogen, carotid luminal diameter, etc.)?

For review articles:

1. Were explicit, systematic methods used to determine and assess the articles reviewed? If this is a systematic review, were the methods of review explicitly expressed?
2. Does the reviewer have biases related to his or her own research and publication or links to pharmaceutical or medical equipment manufacturers that may sway the review?

In neurology, evidence is just as important as it is in other areas. At times using EBM approaches in neurology creates problems that should at least be recognized.

1. Rare diseases are common neurology, and rare diseases may be difficult to study using randomized trials design because large numbers of patients may be hard to come by.
2. Outcome measures may be soft in some areas of neurology with slowly developing change (e.g., progression in multiple sclerosis, worsening in Alzheimer disease) so that surrogate markers such as MRI or cognitive testing are used, which may or may not express meaningful changes in disease outcomes.
3. Time constraints in acute neurologic disease may mean that only a small sample of a population at risk can enter studies,

threatening the generalizability and utility of treatments based on such a population (e.g., acute stroke trials).

Having said this, many of the new treatments referenced in this text are based on sound clinical trials methodology and will, it is hoped, stand up to the test of time. Where possible we have referenced levels of evidence or grades of recommendation using the Oxford Center for Evidence-Based Medicine guidelines for such grading (Table 36.1). We have also tried to reference where the evidence is lacking in an area of treatment.

A note about ARR, RRR, and NNT, and their use in neurology: A key element assessing whether a treatment is "worthwhile" even if it is statistically better than the comparator is the absolute risk reduction (ARR) of the treatment, which can also be expressed as a number needed to treat (NNT). The ARR is the absolute difference in event rates of an adverse event of interest between the control group and treatment group. It is expressed arithmetically as the absolute value of the event rate in the treatment group minus the event rate in the comparison group. For example, if there are 10% strokes in the control group and 5% in the treatment group, the absolute risk reduction is 5%.

Such results are often expressed as relative risk reduction (RRR), which is the proportion of adverse events that would have occurred in the control group avoided by the treatment. In the example given above, the RRR would be 100%. Pharmaceutical reports often emphasize RRR, which sounds larger than ARR but may falsely express the absolute risk reduction, which is after all the "bang for the buck" of treatment.

Another way of expressing the absolute risk reduction is by using number needed to treat (NNT). This is the inverse of the ARR. For example, with an absolute risk reduction of 5%, one needs to treat 20 people to avoid one adverse outcome (1/ARR). With an absolute risk reduction of 1%, one would need to treat 100 people to avoid the outcome. NNT is a useful measure of clinical utility.

GLOSSARY OF EVIDENCE-BASED MEDICINE TERMS

Absolute risk reduction: the absolute difference in event rates of an adverse event of interest between the control group and treatment group.

Blinding: any one of the patients, clinicians, pharmacy staff, technicians, assessors, and so on can be blinded (multiple levels of blinding).

TABLE 36.1. Oxford Centre for Evidence-based Medicine Levels of Evidence (May 2001)

Level	Therapy/Prevention, Aetiology/Harm	Prognosis	Diagnosis	Differential Diagnosis/ Symptom Prevalence Study	Economic and Decision Analyses
1a	SR (with homogeneity*) of RCTs	SR (with homogeneity*) of inception cohort studies; CDR† validated in different populations	SR (with homogeneity*) of Level 1 diagnostic studies; CDR† with 1b studies from different clinical centers	SR (with homogeneity*) of prospective cohort studies	SR (with homogeneity*) of Level 1 economic studies
1b	Individual RCT (with narrow Confidence Interval‡)	Individual inception cohort study with ≥80% follow-up; CDR† validated in a single population	Validating** cohort study with good††† reference standards; or CDR† tested within one clinical center	Prospective cohort study with good follow-up****	Analysis based on clinically sensible costs or alternatives; systematic review(s) of the evidence; and including multi-way sensitivity analyses
1c	All or none§	All or none case-series	Absolute SpPins and SnNouts††	All or none case-series	Absolute better-value or worse-value analyses ††††
2a	SR (with homogeneity*) of cohort studies	SR (with homogeneity*) of either retrospective cohort studies or untreated control groups in RCTs	SR (with homogeneity*) of Level >2 diagnostic studies	SR (with homogeneity*) of 2b and better studies	SR (with homogeneity*) of Level >2 economic studies
2b	Individual cohort study (including low quality RCT; e.g., <80% follow-up)	Retrospective cohort study or follow-up of untreated control patients in an RCT; Derivation of CDR† or validated on split-sample§§§ only	Exploratory** cohort study with good††† reference standards; CDR† after derivation, or validated only on split-sample§§§ or databases	Retrospective cohort study, or poor follow-up	Analysis based on clinically sensible costs or alternatives; limited review(s) of the evidence, or single studies; and including multi-way sensitivity analyses
2c	"Outcomes" Research; Ecological studies	"Outcomes" Research		Ecological studies	Audit or outcomes research
3a	SR (with homogeneity*) of case-control studies		SR (with homogeneity*) of 3b and better studies	SR (with homogeneity*) of 3b and better studies	SR (with homogeneity*) of 3b and better studies
3b	Individual Case-Control Study		Non-consecutive study; or without consistently applied reference standards	Non-consecutive cohort study, or very limited population	Analysis based on limited alternatives or costs, poor quality estimates of data, but including sensitivity analyses incorporating clinically sensible variations
4	Case-series (and poor quality cohort and case-control studies§§)	Case-series (and poor quality prognostic cohort studies***)	Case-control study, poor or non-independent reference standard	Case-series or superseded reference standards	Analysis with no sensitivity analysis
5	Expert opinion without explicit critical appraisal, or based on physiology, bench research or "first principles"	Expert opinion without explicit critical appraisal, or based on physiology, bench research or "first principles"	Expert opinion without explicit critical appraisal, or based on physiology, bench research or "first principles"	Expert opinion without explicit critical appraisal, or based on physiology, bench research or "first principles"	Expert opinion without explicit critical appraisal, or based on economic theory or "first principles"

TABLE 36.1. Oxford Centre for Evidence-based Medicine Levels of Evidence (May 2001) (Continued)

Notes

Users can add a minus-sign "−" to denote the level of that fails to provide a conclusive answer because of:

- EITHER a single result with a wide Confidence Interval (such that, for example, an ARR in an RCT is not statistically significant but whose confidence intervals fail to exclude clinically important benefit or harm)
- OR a systematic Review with troublesome (and statistically significant) heterogeneity.
- Such evidence is inconclusive, and therefore can only generate Grade D recommendations.

† By homogeneity we mean a systematic review that is free of worrisome variations (heterogeneity) in the directions and degrees of results between individual studies. Not all systematic reviews with statistically significant heterogeneity need be worrisome, and not all worrisome heterogeneity need be statistically significant. As noted above, studies displaying worrisome heterogeneity should be tagged with a "−" at the end of their designated level.

‡ Clinical Decision Rule. (These are algorithms or scoring systems which lead to a prognostic estimation or a diagnostic category.)

§ See note #2 for advice on how to understand, rate and use trials or other studies with wide confidence intervals.

§§ Met when all patients died before the Rx became available, but some now survive on it; or when some patients died before the Rx became available, but none now die on it.

§§§ By poor quality cohort study we mean one that failed to clearly define comparison groups and/or failed to measure exposures and outcomes in the same (preferably blinded), objective way in both exposed and non-exposed individuals and/or failed to identify or appropriately control known confounders and/or failed to carry out a sufficiently long and complete follow-up of patients. By poor quality case-control study we mean one that failed to clearly define comparison groups and/or failed to measure exposures and outcomes in the same (preferably blinded), objective way in both cases and controls and/or failed to identify or appropriately control known confounders.

§§§§ Split-sample validation is achieved by collecting all the information in a single tranche, then artificially dividing this into "derivation" and "validation" samples.

†† An "Absolute SpPin" is a diagnostic finding whose Specificity is so high that a Positive result rules-in the diagnosis. An "Absolute SnNout" is a diagnostic finding whose Sensitivity is so high that a Negative result rules-out the diagnosis.

‡‡ Good, better, bad and worse refer to the comparisons between treatments in terms of their clinical risks and benefits.

††† Good reference standards are independent of the test, and applied blindly or objectively to applied to all patients. Poor reference standards are haphazardly applied, but still independent of the test. Use of a non-independent reference standard (where the 'test' is included in the 'reference', or where the 'testing' affects the 'reference') implies a level 4 study.

†††† Better-value treatments are clearly as good but cheaper, or better at the same or reduced cost. Worse-value treatments are as good and equally or worse and equally or worse and more expensive.

** Validating studies test the quality of a specific diagnostic test, based on prior evidence. An exploratory study collects information and trawls the data (e.g. using a regression analysis) to find which factors are 'significant'.

*** By poor quality prognostic cohort study we mean one in which sampling was biased in favour of patients who already had the target outcome, or the measurement of outcomes was accomplished in <80% of study patients, or outcomes were determined in an unblinded, non-objective way, or there was no correction for confounding factors.

**** Good follow-up in a differential diagnosis study is >80%, with adequate time for alternative diagnoses to emerge (e.g., 1−6 months acute, 1−5 years chronic)

Grades of Recommendation

A consistent level 1 studies

B consistent level 2 or 3 studies or extrapolations from level 1 studies

C level 4 studies or extrapolations from level 2 or 3 studies

D level 5 evidence or troublingly inconsistent or inconclusive studies of any level

"Extrapolations" are where data are used in a situation which has potentially clinically important differences than the original study situation.

Produced by Bob Phillips, Chris Ball, Dave Sackett, Doug Badenoch, Sharon Straus, Brian Haynes, Martin Dawes since November 1998.

Reproduced with permission, 2007

Blinding means that some or all of these individuals were unaware of which study group the patient was entered into.

Concealed allocation: adequate measures to hide study group assignments from those who are responsible for placing the patient in the trial (for example, sealed envelopes, central allocation, coded bottles).

Confidence interval: this is a measure of the range of values within which it can be relatively sure that the true value for the whole population lies (usually measured at the 95% CI level).

Intention to treat: in this study design all patients allocated to a treatment arm, whether or not they got that treatment, are analyzed statistically in that arm and not switched out of it.

Number needed to treat: the NNT is the number of patients that need to be treated to prevent one adverse outcome. It is 1/ARR.

Relative risk reduction: the proportion of adverse events in the control group that are avoided in the treatment group.

Sensitivity: the proportion of people with target disease or disorder who have a positive test.

Specificity: the proportion of people without the target disease who have a negative test.

Systematic review: this is a review of a topic where the methods of the review are explicitly stated and aimed to systematically review all the literature on a topic, published, and if possible, unpublished. Usually there are two reviewers who independently come to a determination about the strength of the literature and what the literature indicates about a topic. Often reviews of treatment or surgical procedures.

Suggested Readings

www.cebm.net The Oxford Center for Evidence-Based Medicine has extensive tutorials and information related to evidence-based medicine including useful downloads and tables.

www.cche.net The Centre for Health Evidence at the University of Alberta has an extensive collection of tutorials and information about EBM.

Bussière M, Wiebe S. The numbers needed to treat for neurological disorders. *Can J Neurol Sci*. 2005;32(4):440–449.

Coyle PK. Evidence-based medicine and clinical trials. *Neurology*. 200;68(suppl):S3–S7.

Index

Note: Page numbers followed by *f* or *t* denote figure or tables, respectively.

Glossary of Common Neurologic Terms

Much of medical education is concerned with learning "medicalese," the medical terms for various signs, symptoms, diseases, findings, or other medical phenomena. It is a good habit to use common language as much as possible and avoid the trap of using "medicalese" too extensively. It is better to describe in common language your observations of a patient's exam or behavior rather than overinterpreting it unless you are sure you are correct. The physiology never lies; language frequently obscures meaning. The following terms are found commonly in neurology and are worth understanding.

Note that this glossary includes basic terms used frequently in neurology and is not meant to be exhaustive. In addition, eponyms (names used to describe a sign, symptom, disease, or other medical phenomenon) are not defined and should be sought in the index. Most anatomic terms will be found in the text and will not be referred to here unless they are very common.

A- : lack of

Ab- : away from

Ad- : towards

Abulia: lack of interest in activities, usually due to frontal lobe disease

Acalculia: difficulty calculating

Acquired: occurring sometime after birth, later in life

Acute: sudden

Agnosagnosia: denial or lack of awareness of a neurologic deficit

Agnosia: disorder of recognition of objects or people not due to loss of a primary sensory function. For example, visual agnosia, inability to recognize objects by vision where vision is otherwise preserved

Agraphia: inability to write

Alexia: inability to read

Amaurosis: visual loss

Anomia: difficult naming

Apraxia: A condition in which the patient understands the task, is willing to do it, has the motor and sensory capacity to do it, but is unable to perform the activity

Aprosody: loss of the melodic or emotional content of speech or understanding of these factors in the speech of others

Areflexia: lack of one or more reflexes

Asterixis: a sudden relaxation of muscle activity lasting a few hundred milliseconds, usually seen in the arms, related to metabolic encephalopathy

Ataxia: refers to the presence of incoordination. Can refer to gait, limb function, truncal stability, speech, respiration, or other movements

Athetosis: writhing, slow, abnormal movements. Sometimes combined with chorea

Aura: pertaining to migraine, neurologic symptoms accompanying migraine. Pertaining to seizures, a focal seizure that the patient senses in some way (e.g., rising sensation, odd smell) that may progress to a more generalized seizure

Autonomic: the part of the nervous system that is usually "unconscious," serving functions such as gut motility, voiding, pupil response, heart rate, sweating, and so on.

Axon: the major nerve fiber leading away from the nerve cell

Basal ganglia: the deep portions of the brain including the caudate, putamen, globus pallidus, thalamus, and smaller basal ganglia nuclei

Brainstem: the part of the brain at the base of the brain including the midbrain, pons, and medulla

Bruit: sound heard over a vessel (e.g. Carotid bruit.)

Buccal-oral apraxia: inability to make movement to command with the mouth and lips

Cauda equina: literally, horse's tail. The nerve roots that emerge from the base of the spinal cord serving the legs and the genitalia

Cerebellum: organ at the base of the brain that is involved in coordination and programming of motor activity

Cerebral: pertaining to the cerebrum, the brain

Chorea: abnormal jerky, arrhythmic movement of limbs or body. Sometimes combines with athetosis (choreoathetosis)

Circumlocutions: literally, speaking around a word. Where a patient will define a word but be unable to name the word itself

Clonic: rhythmic jerking

Coma: a state where a patient is "not awake, and not asleep." A pathological state where there is no visible sign of awareness of the environment, but not "locked-in," in which a patient is aware but unable to signal that awareness to examiners

Congenital: occurring at or before birth

Contralateral: on the opposite side

Convulsion: a tonic-clonic seizure

Cortical: pertaining to the surface of the newer cortex of the brain (neocortex), usually gray matter

Corticobulbar: the pathway connecting the cortex with the muscles of speech and swallowing

Delirium: a subacute alteration of attention, consciousness, and orientation usually associated with agitation and autonomic signs, often due to a medical illness or a withdrawal state

Dementia: a progressive state over more than 6 months with decline in multiple areas of cognitive function

Dendrite: small branching extensions from the nerve cell body, which usually receive information via synapses from other nerve cells

Diplopia: having double vision

Diploplia: a malapropism, common to residents in training. There is no such medical term. It's *diplopia*.

Distal: referring to further away from the center of the body or further away from the origin of a structure. For example, distal ulnar nerve, further down the arm or hand from the origin of the ulnar nerve in the brachial plexus

Dizziness: this is not a medical term. When the patient speaks of dizziness, they must be asked to define what the sensation is in other words

Dura: the thick membrane that surrounds the brain, it is outside of the arachnoid and pial membranes that cover the brain

Dys- : refers to something being abnormal, for example, dysfunction, abnormal function. A frequently "dysused" word

Dysarthria: slurred speech without problems with language production

Dysdiadochokinesis: a wonderful, fairly useless term that describes arrhythmic supination and pronation movements of the forearm, usually in patients with cerebellar disease

Dysmetria: abnormal measurement of movement

Dysphagia: abnormal swallowing

Dystonia: refers to abnormal increased tone that is either focal or generalized

Embolism: refers to the migration of something (air, clot, fat, etc.) downstream in a blood vessel to another area, sometimes causing infarction

Encephalitis: infection or inflammation of the brain substance

Encephalopathy: a general disorder of cognition, usually acute, with altered attention and alertness

Epidural: outside the dura

Epilepsy: the state of having repeated unprecipitated seizures

Exacerbation: a worsening of something

Extinction: When a patient notices stimuli only from one side when stimulated on both sides simultaneously. Assumes that sensation is intact

Extrapyramidal: Relating to neural pathways situated outside or independent of the pyramidal tracts

Fascicle: literally, a bundle, usually referring to a nerve fiber tract

Fasciculation: a twitching movement in a muscle caused by abnormal firing of a single lower motor neuron

Fibrillation: abnormal independent firing of a muscle fiber visible only on electromyography, not visible clinically

Fortification: usually referring to a fortification spectra, a zig-zag visual aura associated with migraine that looks somewhat like a fortress

Fundus: the back of the eye. Plural: fundi

Grand mal: an obsolete term for generalized seizures

Graphesthesia: ability to determine the identity of a number drawn on the hand

Hemianopia: loss of vision in one visual field. Usually homonymous (both visual fields on one side affected) or bitemporal (both lateral [temporal] visual fields affected)

Hemiparesis: weakness of one side that is incomplete

Hemiplegia: weakness of one side that is complete

Hydrocephalus: literally, water on the brain, increased fluid in the ventricles of the brain. May be communicating or obstructive

Hyper- : too much

Hypo- : too little

Iatrogenic: something caused by what doctors do, a medical misadventure

Ictal: usually pertaining to a seizure. Thus, interictal = between seizures, postictal = after a seizure

Idiopathic: meaning doctors don't know why something happens to someone. For example, idiopathic epilepsy, without a known cause

Infarction: death of a tissue due to lack of oxygenation, usually from lack of blood flow

Insult: while in other fields one might take offense, in neurology this means some kind of injury

Intraaxial: inside of the central nervous system

Ipsilateral: on the same side

Lacune: a small vascular lesion deep in the brain commonly seen in patients with hypertension or diabetes

Lamination: in neurology, refers to the fact that certain motor or sensory tracts are organized in layers with different parts of the tract going to different areas in an organized fashion

Lateral: to one side

Lesion: a non-specific term that refers either to an area of abnormality (e.g., lesions in multiple sclerosis) or some kind of injury otherwise unspecified (i.e., ulnar nerve lesion)

Malacia: a softening, such as encephalomalacia after trauma

Medial: towards the midline

Meningitis: infection or inflammation in the spinal fluid compartment

Mesial: in the midline, for example mesial cortex, the most midline of the cortices

Mutism: being unable to speak

Myelo- : referring to the spinal cord

Myoclonus: rapid, jerky muscle movements in one or more muscle groups. (When in multiple groups, referred to as multifocal myoclonus.)

Myopathy: a muscle disorder

Myotonia: an altered muscle tone

Neglect: when a patient ignores stimuli (visual, tactile, etc.) from one side of the body or space

Neologisms: literally, the making of new words, refers usually to abnormal language production in aphasic patients

Neuraxis: the entirety of the nervous system. Also refers to a Canadian death metal band

Neuron: a nerve cell

Neuropathy: a nerve disorder. Usually refers to a peripheral nervous system or cranial nerve disorder

Nystagmus: abnormal, rhythmic eye movements that are either pendular (same velocity in both directions) or jerk (having a fast and a slow phase)

Obtundation: this is a term commonly used by medical residents that has no medical meaning and should be avoided at all costs

Occlusion: complete blockage, as opposed to stenosis.

-opathy: a disorder of something. (e.g., neuropathy, myelopathy)

Palsy: a persistent injury, such as a radial nerve palsy. A delightfully antique term

Papilledema: swollen disc margins in the fundi due to increased intracranial pressure

Paralysis: loss of the ability to move something, may be focal or generalized

Paraphasia: errors of word or syllable choice

Paraplegia: bilateral complete leg weakness

Parasomnia: abnormal behavior or movement during sleep

Paresthesia: abnormal sensation, usually uncomfortable, such as tingling

Paroxysmal: occurring suddenly, usually transiently

Petit mal: an archaic term, literally, "small bad." Instead use *absence seizure*

Plaque: specific term in neurology not referring to dental hygiene, but to an area of demyelination in the central nervous system

Proximal: referring usually to nearer to the center of the body, rather than distal, further away from the center of the body. Or nearer to the beginning of a structure, such as proximal carotid artery

Pyramidal: the corticospinal tract. The term refers to the pyramids of the medulla where the corticospinal tract crosses the midline

Radical: referring to a nerve root, not a counter-culture rebel. As in radiculopathy, something wrong with a nerve root

Reflex: usually a neurologic phenomenon where stimulating a nerve causes a programmed reaction, such as the knee jerk response

Seizure: a transient neurologic phenomenon caused by sudden abnormal firing of a group of cerebral neurons

Spasticity: an abnormal increase in tone, usually due to problems with the upper motor neuron

Stenosis: a narrowing or partial blockage. For example, spinal stenosis

Stereognosis: ability to identify objects using the sense of touch

Stroke: sudden neurologic deficit due to vascular disease

Subarachnoid: under the arachnoid membrane, above the pial membrane, outside of the brain

Subdural: under the dura

Supratentorial: literally, above the tentorium. The neocortex and diencephalon

Synapse: a connection between two neurons

Syncope: a sudden loss of consciousness, usually transient, due to reduced cerebral perfusion

Tardive: delayed or late

Thrombus: a blood clot forming in one place and staying there (e.g., deep vein thrombosis)

Tinnitus: a ringing sound that either just the patient (subjective) or observers and the patient (objective) can hear. Can be pulsatile or continuous

Tonic: a stiffening

Tract: nerves that travel together, usually serving a similar function (e.g. spinothalamic tract, which observes pin and temperature sensation)

TIA: transient ischemic attack, a temporary focal deficit due to vascular disease, usually less than 30 minutes. Other terms such as RIND and stroke in evolution have no specific meaning and are no longer used

Tremor: a rhythmic movement of part or all of the body

Vertigo: a perception of self or environmental spin